THE WHOLE
BODY
TONE UP
BOOK

by Valerie Hockert

Exercises
That Really Work
to Trim and Tone
Your Body!

Valerie Hockert
Wholebodytoneup@aol.com

Author's Note

For the past many years I have taught courses in exercise. During that time I've come to realize that many people require a comprehensive exercise program that treats the whole body. Even people who participate in slymnastics or sports are not guaranteed a workout for the entire system. So I devised the Whole Body Tone Up Program.

This program consists of over 100 exercises, including jogging and rope jumping with a smathering of weight lifting included. Some of these exercises are used for warmups in dance; some are poses used in yoga and others are exercises used in physical therapy. Together they comprise a diverse, highly effective exercise plan.

If you've decided to get in shape, there's no better time to begin this program. It will not only help in controlling weight, but a faithfully followed exercise program will always yield a feeling of fitness and vitality.

Exercise is a great aid for weight control. If you have decided to get in shape, now is the time to begin and this is the book for you. An excellent program basically designed with you in mind.

Contents

Caution: When you begin any new exercise program, remember to use moderation and work *gradually* toward the more strenuous exercises. It is recommended that you see your physician before beginning any new exercise program.

Introduction

Physical fitness is a measure of your body's strength, endurance, agility and coordination. Whether you are physically fit or not, can reflect both in your physical body, and your mental/emotional body.

Results from a faithfully followed exercise program can be dramatic--well worth every stretch and grimace. The greatest investment is determination and the returns are many. Some of the numerous benefits from exercising are: better appearance; more strength and coordination; fewer minor aches and stiffness, less fatigue and, one of the most popular effects--it aids in weight control (That is, if you don't end up in the kitchen after every exercise session!)

The main section of the "Whole Body Tone Up Book" includes 100 exercises. It is designed as a comprehensive exercise program. By doing the entire program, you exercise your entire body, and will see the greatest benefits.

If you're more interested in spot exercises, there are specific sections in the book for the waist, stomach, thighs and back. And for those with great expectations but limited time, there's a "crash course" at the end of the book.

Go through as many exercises as you can if you're doing the longer section; even though you may not be able to complete all of them the first few times. It's best to start at the beginning each day with at least half hour sessions, if possible.

Go through the whole section each time if you're doing the section for spot exercising. Do each exercise six times in the beginning and work up to 20. (If you're more ambitious than that--go for it!) Start at the beginning of each section each time because the easier ones are first and it will help you prepare for the succeeding exercises.

If you have a heart or respiratory condition, check with your doctor before beginning these exercises. This is also advisable if you're over 30 and have not had a recent checkup.

Exercising regularly requires determination, but the benefits are so fantastic! After a very short time, you'll not only look better, but you'll feel like you have more energy. Hang in there--and happy exercising!

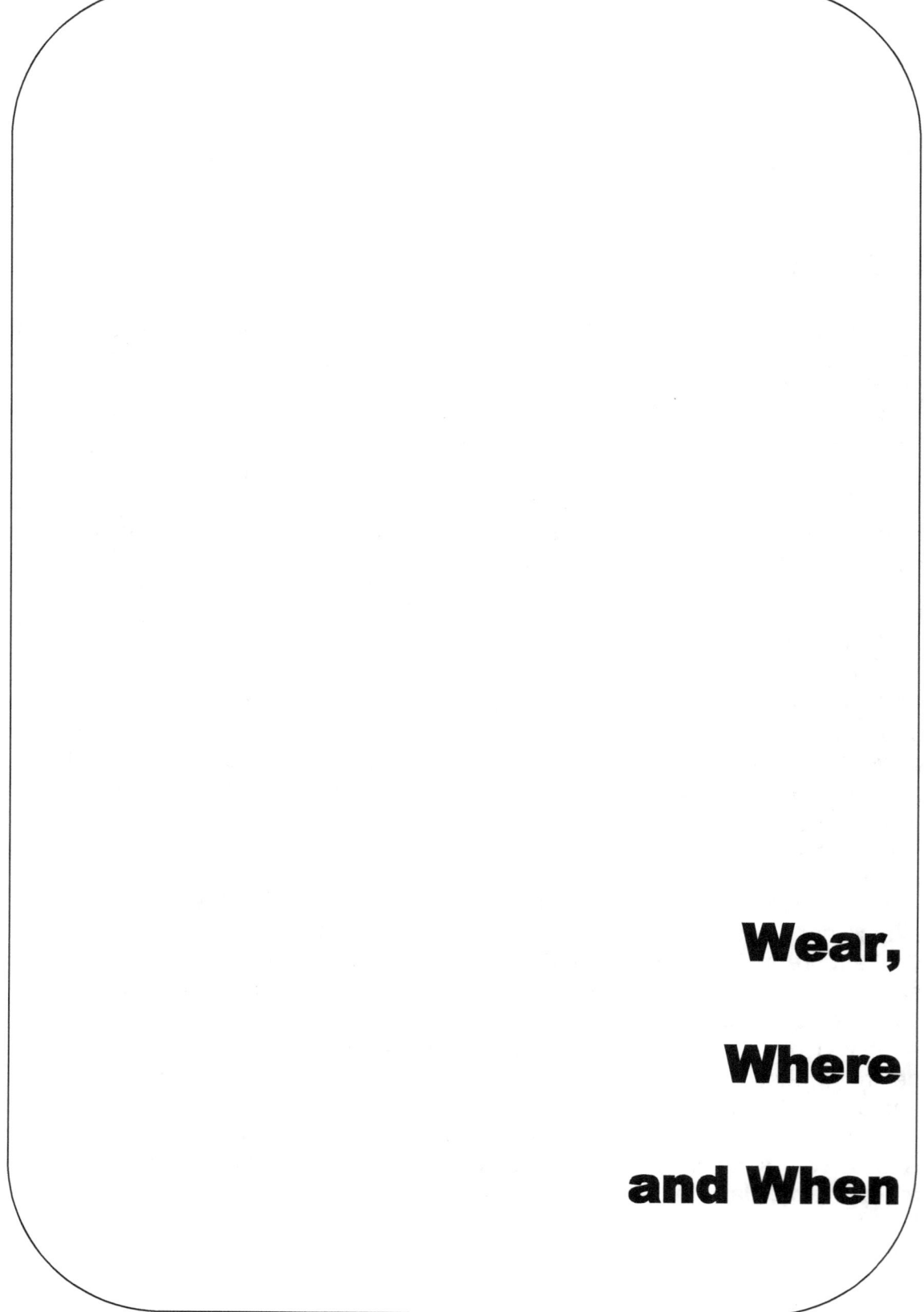

Wear,

Where

and When

(Make It Easy On Yourself....)

Wear something loose and comfortable that will not get in your way, like a sweatsuit, leotards or jogging shorts and a t-shirt. It is important to dress warm enough, because when muscles get cold, they tend to stiffen up.

Find a well-ventilated room for exercising, where you have some space to move around. A carpeted room is ideal. If you are on a hard floor, you may want to use an exercise mat or scatter rug.

Try playing your favorite tunes--it's always more fun to exercise to music. Avoid watching television, though--it makes it harder to concentrate on exercising.

These exercises should be done daily in order to get the optimum effects. At first, you'll probably feel some soreness; that's only because you're out of shape. Keep at it, though, if too much time lapses between exercising, you'll be just as sore the second time around.

I'd suggest doing these exercises at a time during the day when you are not too sleepy. If you're a morning person, early in the day is perfect; otherwise wait until later in the day when it won't be such a struggle for you.

Do the exercises as they are described and illustrated--no cheating! The pulls should be felt according to how vigorously you're exercising. There are two reasons you would not feel the pulls though, either you exercise frequently or you're not doing them correctly. Okay--ready? Let's go....

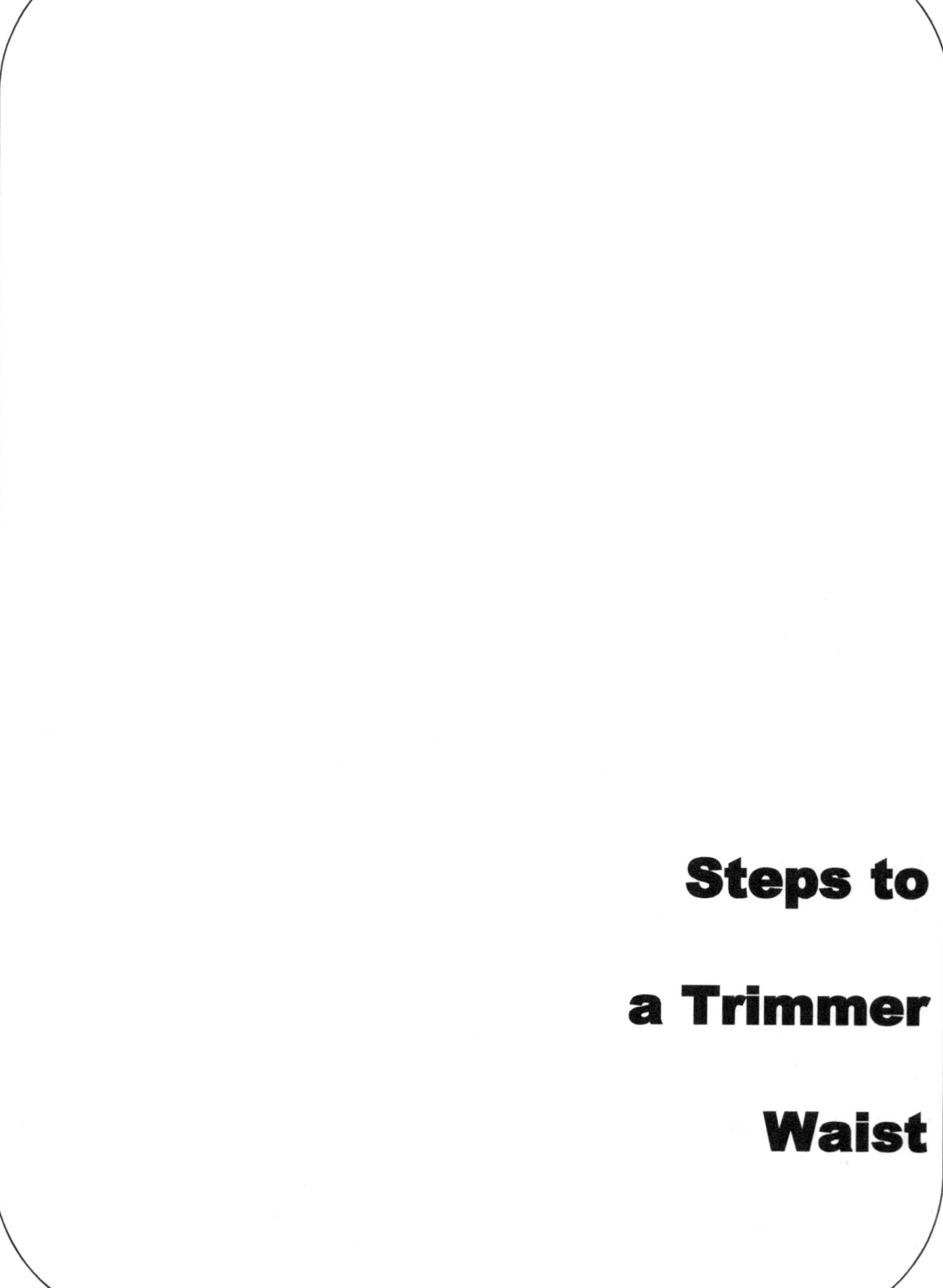

Steps to

a Trimmer

Waist

(Less Is More....)

Sitting Overhead Stretch

Sitting down on the floor, cross your legs "Indian Style," with your back straight. First, with your right hand reach way, way up, as far as you can reach. Then do the same on the left side.

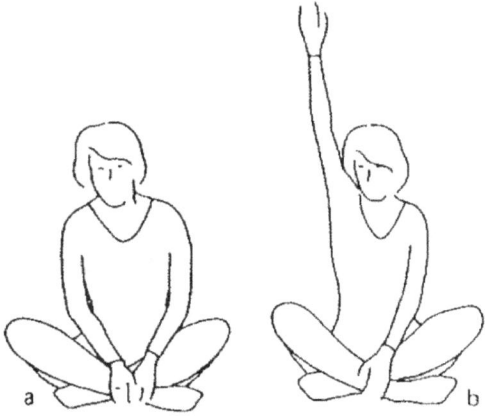

Figure 1

You will fee the pull through the middle. If you can't feel the pull, stretch a little harder. Feel it now? *(Figure 1)*

Sitting Overhead Stretch/Wrist

Still sitting on the floor with your legs crossed, stretch up with your right arm. With the left hand, hold your right wrist and pull down while leaning slightly to the left. Now, stretch up with the left arm. With the right hand, hold your left wrist and pull while leaning slightly to the right.

Again you will feel pull in the side waist area, and also in the arms. *(Figure 2)*

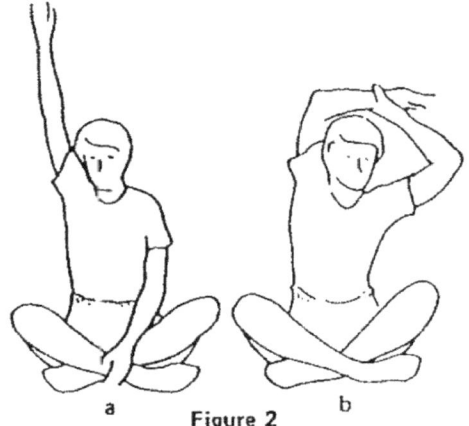

a   Figure 2   b

Sitting Overhead Side Stretch

Sitting in the same position, stretch up and over your head with your right arm. Lean to the left enough to feel a slight pull. Then do the same with your left arm up and over your head and lean to feel a pull. Remember to keep your back straight. Repeat. *(Figure 3)*

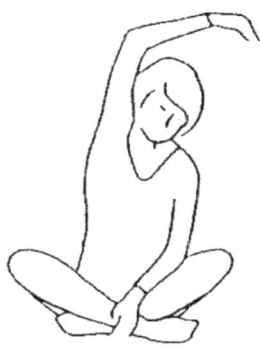

Figure 3

Before starting the next three exercises, let's warm up by sitting with the soles of your feet together. Now hold your feet with your hands. Bring your heels toward you and lean forward at the same time. As you are doing this, try to pull your knees downward without using your hands. Repeat.

Nest, try the same three exercises with the soles of your feet together. They will give the same pulls as before with a little extra through the thighs. (Figure 4)

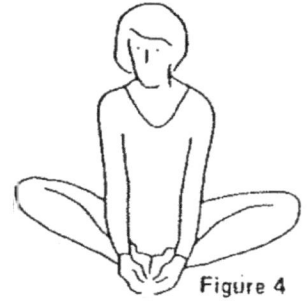

Figure 4

For the next exercise, stand with your feet flat on the floor (except where otherwise indicated), feet spread shoulder width apart keeping your knees straight. The first three are similar to those before, and you should feel the same pulls, particularly through the side, waist and arms. (Figure 5)

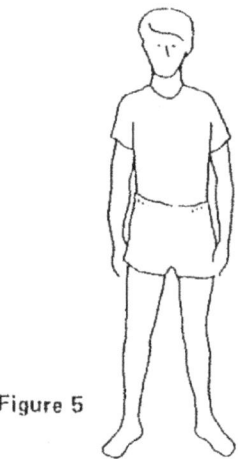

Figure 5

Standing Overhead Stretch

Stretch your right arm up high above your head, reaching with your fingertips as high as you can. Then stretch your left arm up the same way. Repeat.

Standing Overhead Stretch/Wrist

Stretch up with your right arm. With left hand, hold the right wrist and pull down over your head while leaning slightly to the left. Now stretch upward with left arm. With your right hand hold left wrist and pull down while leaning slightly to the right. Repeat, alternating sides.

Standing Overhead Side Stretch

Stretch up and over your head with right arm while leaning slightly to the left. Now stretch over your head with the left arm, while leaning slightly to the right.

Weight Lifting

Use three-pound ladies' dumbbells or five-pound men's dumbbells. If you're really ambitious, use dumbbells with interchangeable weights. Start with the lighter weights and add on.

Arm Pulleys

Standing with a weight in each hand, and keeping feet flat on the floor, reach up *high* with your right arm and pull down with your left arm. You'll be pulling in opposite directions. Now reverse left arm up and right arm down. Repeat. *(Figure 6)*

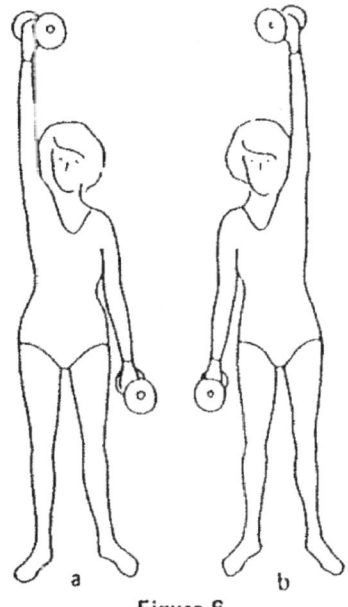

Figure 6

Arm Swing

Standing with weights in your hands, keep your feet flat on the floor and face forward. Put your right arm straight back and your left arm straight forward. Now turn and twist from the waist, so that the left arm is straight back and the right arm is straight forward. Keep your elbows straight. Repeat. *(Figure 7)*

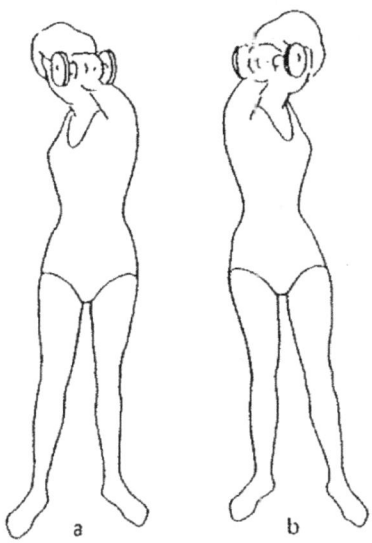

Figure 7

Steps to Flatten Your Stomach

(How to Diminish a Paunchy Profile....)

Some of these exercises to flatten your stomach are also great for trimming the waistline. Usually a large waistline and stomach go together.

For the next three exercises, stand with your feet flat on the floor, spread shoulder width apart, without bending your knees.

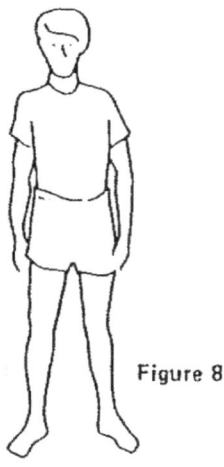

Figure 8

Regular Toe Touch

Touch your toes with the tips of your fingers. Do not bend your knees. *Stretch* up, reaching as high as possible. Repeat. *(Figure 9)*

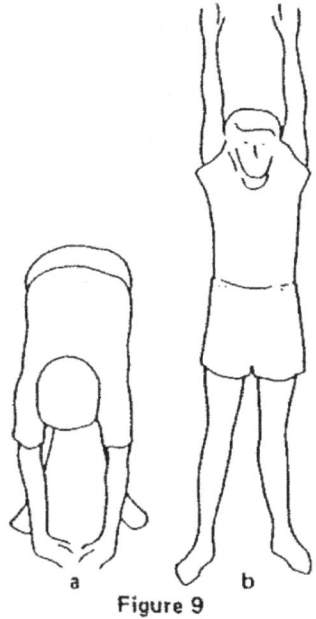

Figure 9

Toe Touch/Hands to Floor

Touch the floor with the palms of your hands. Do not bend your knees. *Stretch* way up with your arms and hands upward. Repeat. *(Figure 10)*

Fan Toe Touch

Stand with your feet spread shoulder width apart and arms outstretched. With your right hand, touch your left toes with the tips of your fingers. Come up and *stretch* with your arms up *high.* Then touch your left hand to your right toes. Again, do *not* bend knees. Repeat.

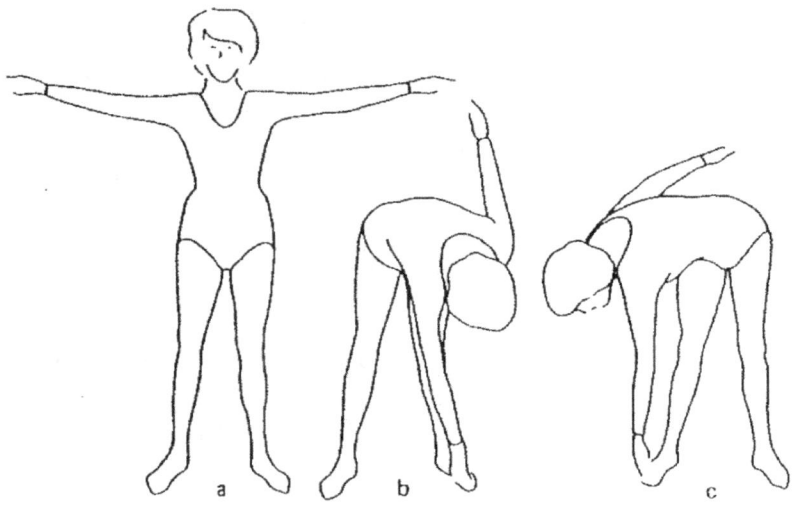

Figure 10

Toe to Toe Swirl

Sit on the floor with your legs stretched in the V-position. Keep your legs stretched as far as possible for greatest results. With both hands on your right foot, turn your head to the right. Swing both hands to the left foot and bring your right arms up over your head. Stretch from the waist by twisting as far around to the right as you can. Alternate and repeat. *(Figure 11)*

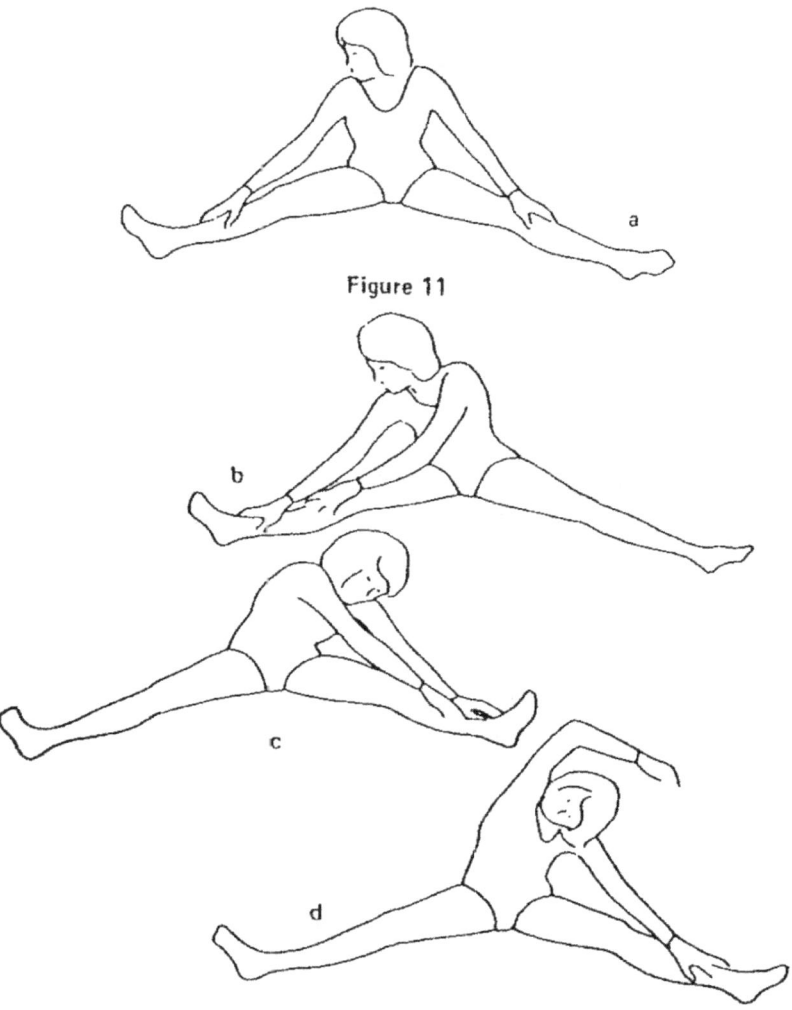

Figure 11

Figure 11 (cont'd.)

V-Turn Pivot

Sitting in the V-stretch position, bring your right foot toward you, and your left foot to the left side. Now turn around to your right, bringing your left arm with you and turning your right shoulder until you see your left foot. *(Figure 12)*

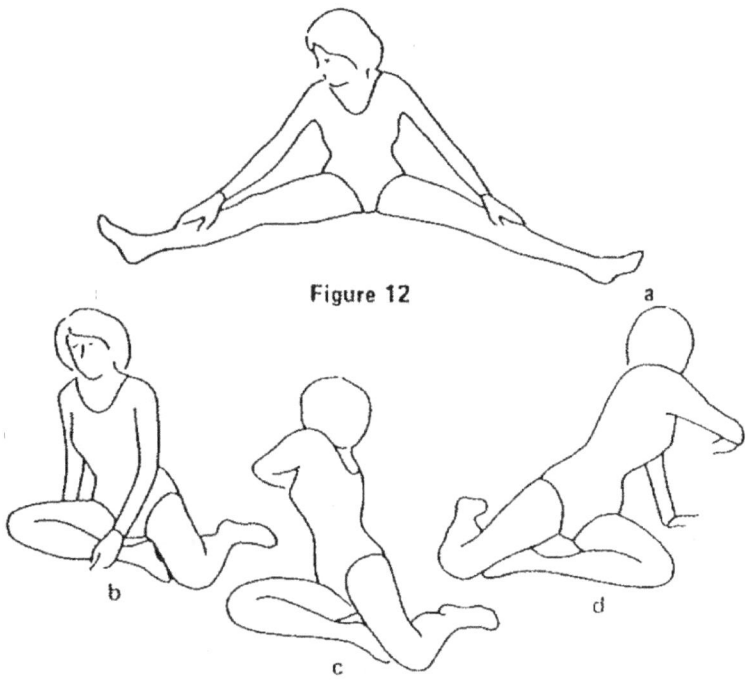

Figure 12

Figure 12 (cont'd.)

For the next five exercises, sit with your legs stretched straight forward and your knees straight.

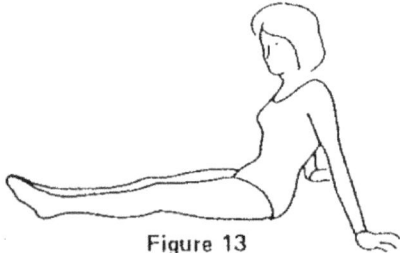

Figure 13

Inch Back

With your arms stretched forward on top of your legs, lean back inch by inch, *slowly* until your lower back is almost touching the floor, but not quite. Then sit up. Do this several times, then go all the way back and stretch your arms straight overhead. Repeat. *(Figure 14)*

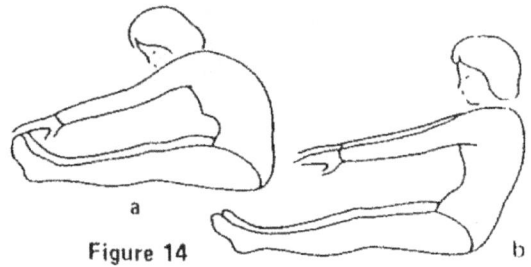

Figure 14

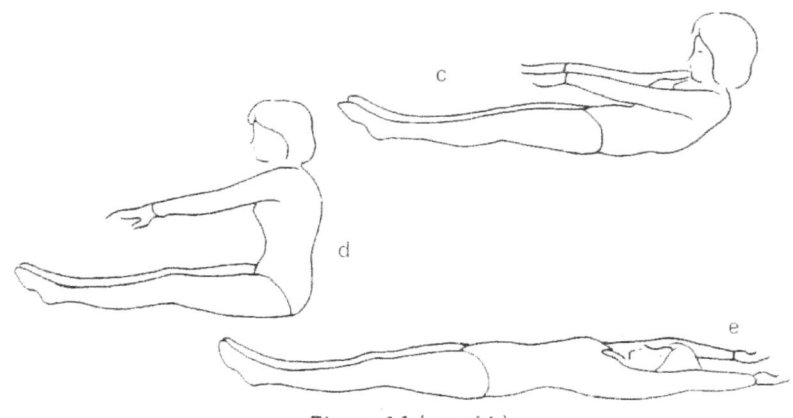

Figure 14 (cont'd.)

Sit Ups

Lie back with your hands stretched straight over your head. Sit up and touch your toes with your hands. Keep your heels on the floor and do not bend your knees.

Fan Sit Ups

Lie back with your hands stretched straight overhead. Sit up and touch the toes on the left foot with your right hand. Then lay back, come up and touch the toes on the right foot with your left hand. Repeat.

Half Sit Ups

Lie back with your arms outstretched. Sit up as far as you can with your lower back still on the floor. Repeat. *(Figure 15)*

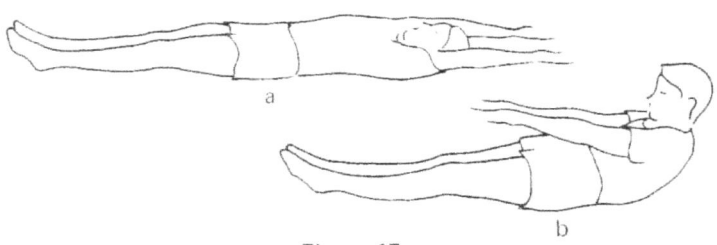

Figure 15

Leg Raiser

Sitting with your legs outstretched, lean back slightly and support yourself by putting your hands on the floor at your sides. First lift your right leg as high as you can, without bending your knees or lifting your buttocks off the floor. Then, the left leg. Now lift both legs at the same time. Lift *high.* Remember--do not bend your knees. You may have to lean back more to do this. (Figure 16)

20

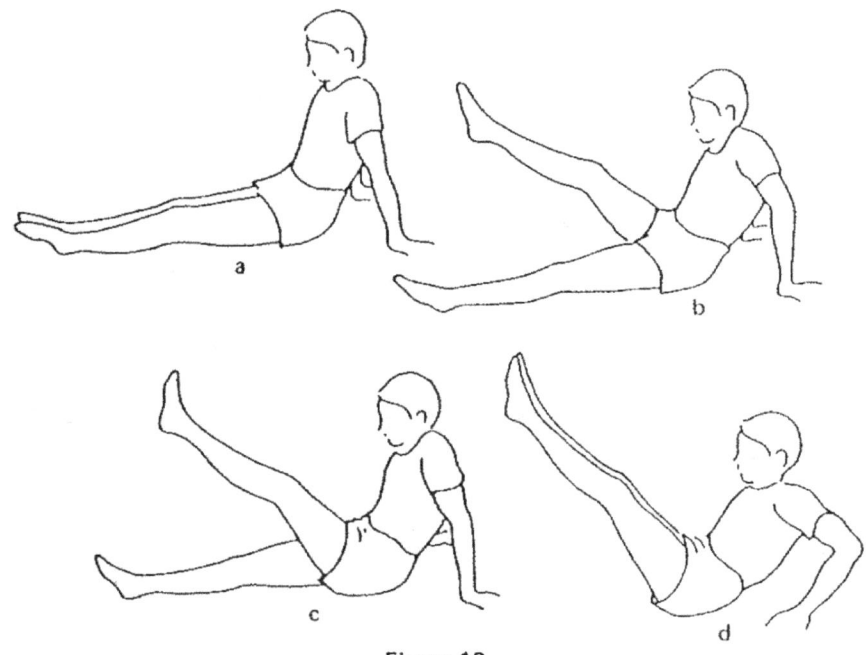

Figure 16

Leg Lift

Now lie flat on your back. Your lower back should be flat on the floor; knees should be bent and slightly apart. Your shoulders should be down, arms outstretched, and palms upward. Bring your right knee toward your chest. Bring your leg up as high as it will go and straighten out your knee. Then lower your leg *slowly* until the leg rests on the floor, keeping your lower back flat on the floor. Now bend your knee up to the starting position. Then do this with your left leg. Repeat. *(Figure 17)*

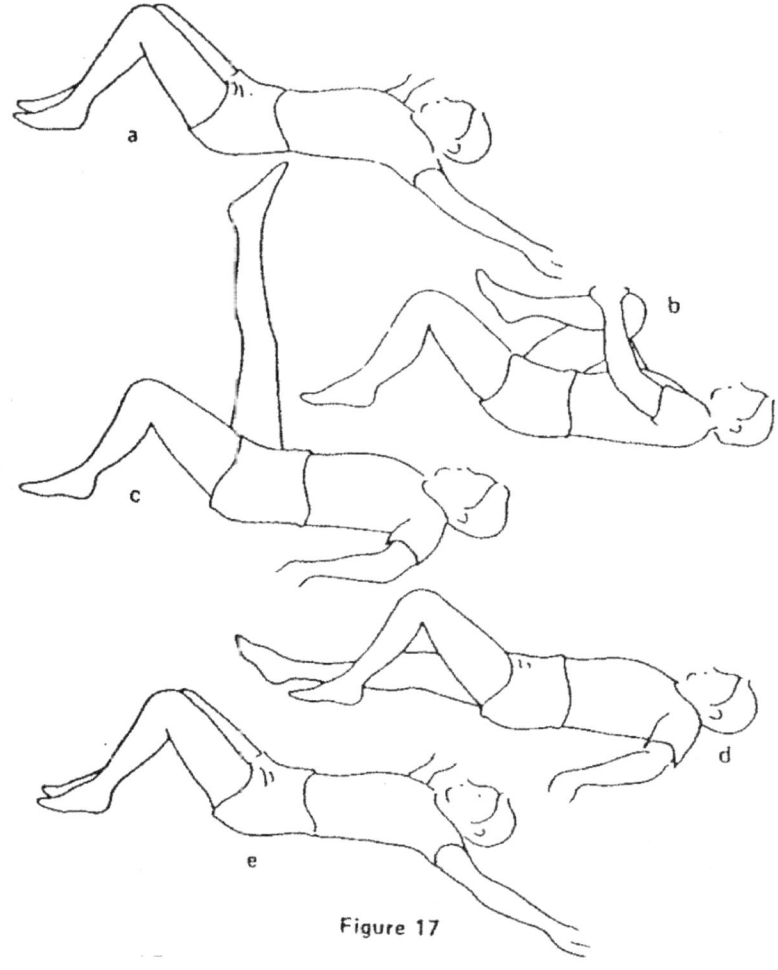

Figure 17

For the next two exercises, lie flat on your stomach.

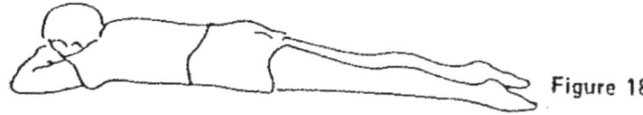

Figure 18

Lift Each Leg, Then Both

Support your chin in your hands. Lift your right leg, keeping your hips on the floor. Then do the same with the left leg. Remember, do not bend your knees. Lift both your legs at the same time. Again, do not bend your knees and keep your hips on the floor. *(Figure 19)*

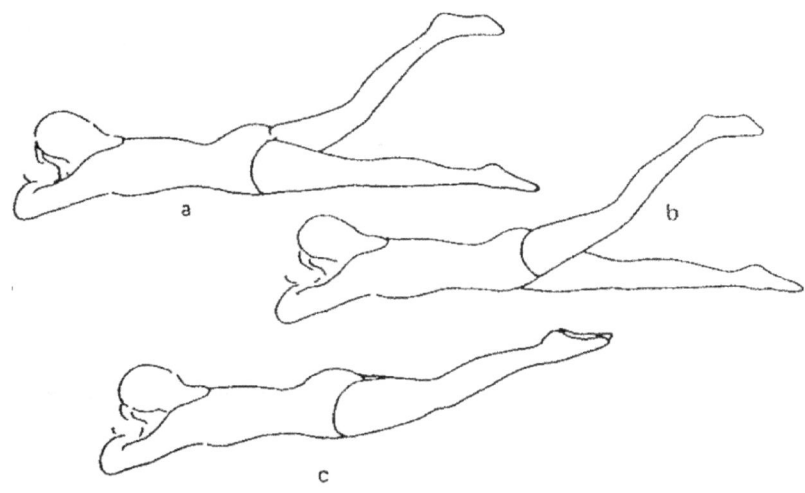

Figure 19

Half Push Ups

Push your hands palm side down on the floor in front of your shoulders. Lift up, keeping hips on the floor. Lower yourself back down to the floor with elbows first, then chest, then chin. *(Figure 20)*

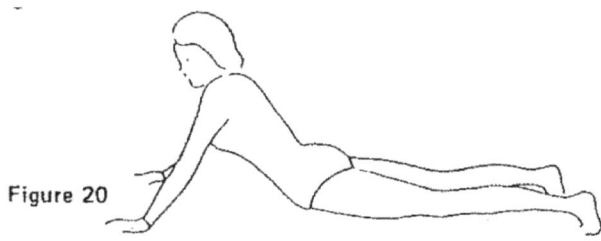

Figure 20

Now get into the straight kneel position for the next two exercises.

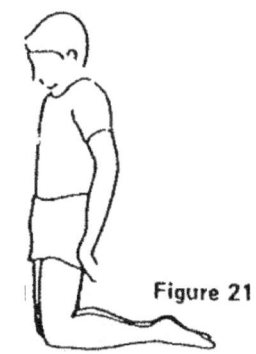

Figure 21

Touch Feet

While kneeling, bend back from the waist and touch your right foot with the right hand; then your left foot with the left hand. *(Figure 22)*

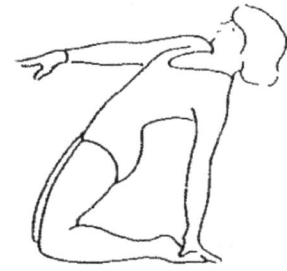

Figure 22

Touch Between Feet

Kneeling, bend back and touch the floor with your right hand between your feet. Do the same with your left hand. *(Figure 23)*

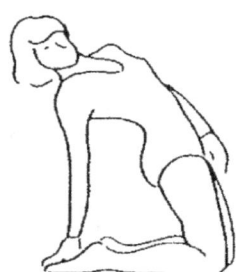

Figure 23

Weight Lifting

Use three-pound ladies' dumbbells or five-pound men's dumbbells. Or, if you're really ambitious, use dumbbells with interchangeable weights. Start with the lighter weights and add on.

Half Sit Ups

With one weight in each hand, lie back with your arms stretched straight above your head. Sit up as far as you can with the lower back still on the floor and bringing your arms up as far as possible. *(Figure 24)*

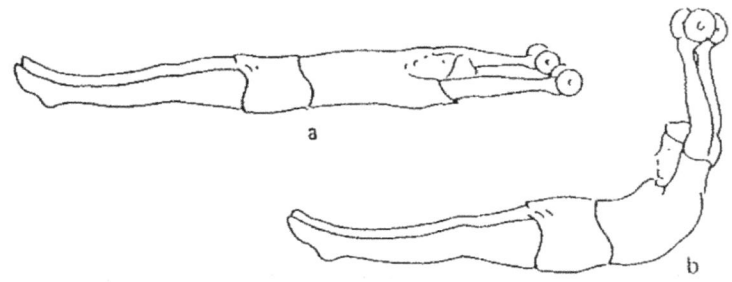

Figure 24

Sit Ups

With one weight in each hand, lie back with your arms stretched overhead. Sit up and touch about an inch above your toes with the weights. Be careful not to drop the weights on your feet. Keep your heels on the floor with your toes pointed forward and remember not to bend your knees. *(Figure 25)*

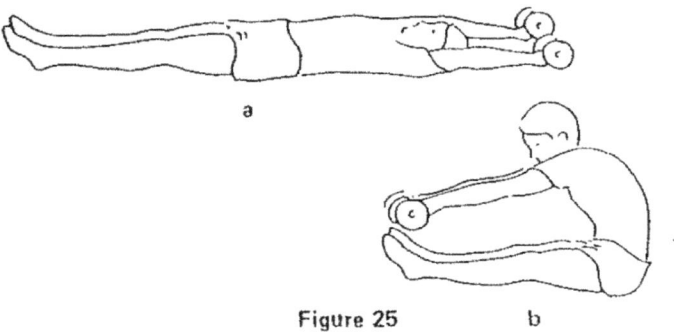

Figure 25   b

Steps to Reduce Your Thighs

(No One's Pulling Your Leg....)

The following exercises are not only great thigh reducers, but they can also help to reduce other areas of your body.

Before starting these next four exercises, let's warm up by sitting with the soles of your feet together. Hold your feet with your hands. Bring your heels toward you and lean forward at the same time. As you are doing this, try to bring your knees down without using your hands. Repeat.

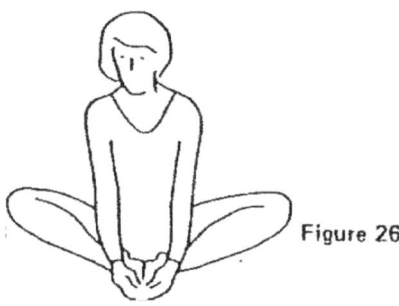

Figure 26

Soles Together Overhead Stretch
With your right hand, stretch upward as high as you can while keeping your left hand on your left knees. Now do the same with the left hand, putting your right hand on your right knee. *(Figure 27)*

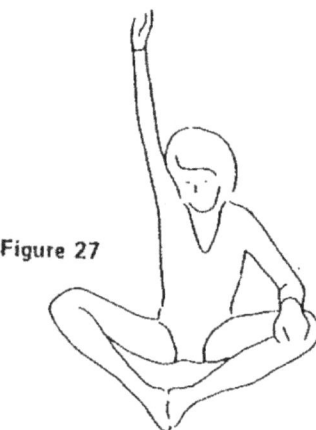

Figure 27

Soles Together Overhead Stretch/Wrist
Stretch up with your right arm. With the left hand, hold your right wrist and pull down toward your head, while slightly leaning to the left. Then alternate sides-- stretch up with your left arm, right hand holds left wrist and pull while leaning slightly to the right. Repeat.

Soles Together Overhead Side Stretch

Reach up and over your head with right arm. Rest your left hand on your feet. Lean to the left just enough to feel a slight pull. Now do the same with the left hand overhead and with the right hand on feet. Repeat.

Soles Together Head to Feet

Sitting with the soles of your feet together, hold your feet with both hands. Then bend forward and *stretch* until your head touches your feet. Remember to sit firmly on the floor. Smile--you're going to like what you see in the mirror! *(Figure 28)*

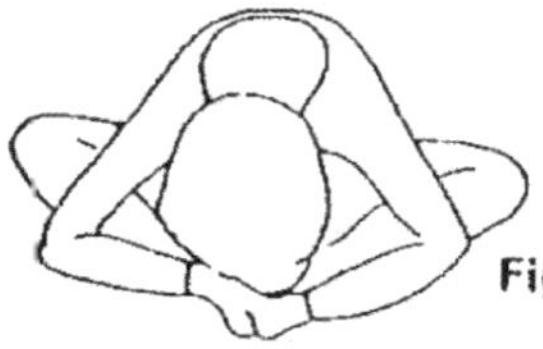

Figure 28

Now stand with your feet flat on the floor, feet spread shoulder width apart without bending your knees.

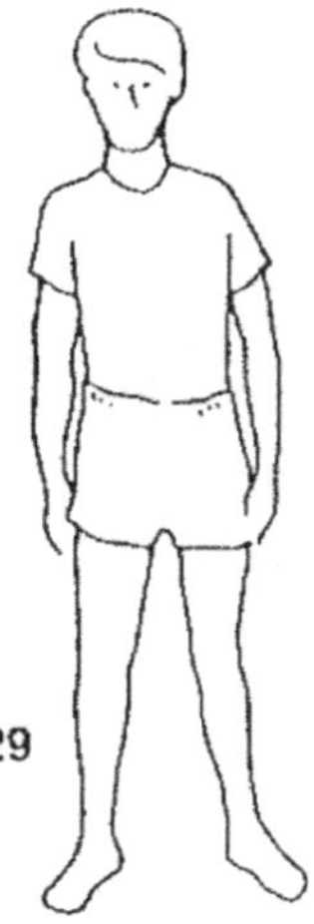

Figure 29

Regular Toe Touch

Touch your toes with the tips of your fingers. Keep your legs straight. Do not bend knees. *Stretch* up, reaching as *high* as possible. Repeat.

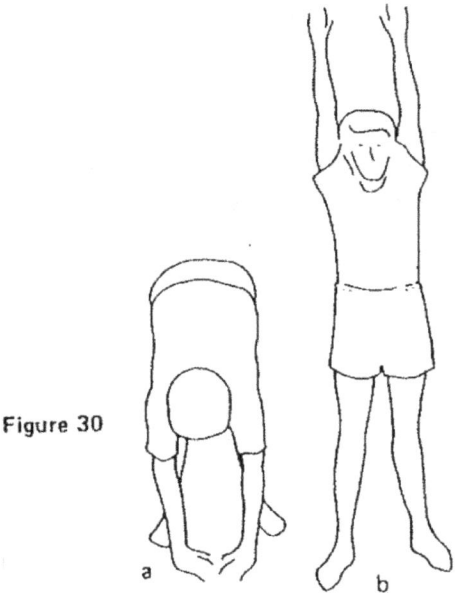

Figure 30

Toe Touch/Hands to Floor

Touch the floor with the palms of your hands without bending your knees. *Stretch* arms overhead with palms up. Repeat *(Figure 30)*

Rag Doll Flop

Touch the floor in front of your toes with the tips of your fingers. Come up about six inches off the floor and then down again. Repeat eight times. Then reach with hands *high* up over your head and repeat the exercise. Remember to keep your knees straight. *(Figure 31)*

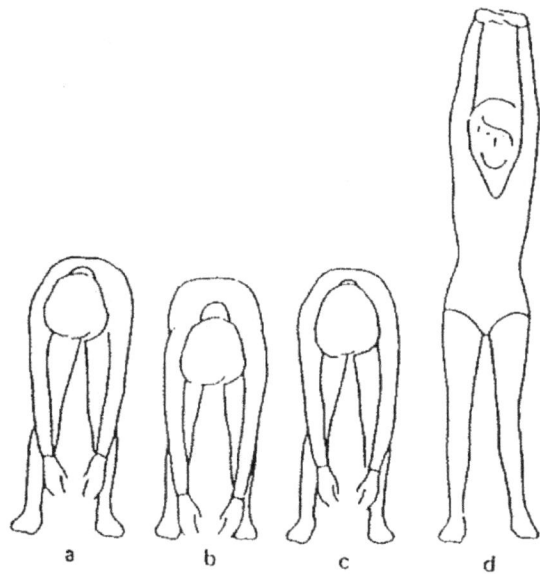

Figure 31

Fan Toe Touch

Stand with your feet spread shoulder width apart and your arms outstretched. With your right hand, touch your left toes. Come up and *stretch* with your arms up *high.* Reverse the exercise so the left hand touches the right toes. Again, do not bend knees. Repeat.

Toe Touch/Clasped Hands

Stand with your feet spread shoulder width apart and your hands clasped. Lift your arms overhead, keeping your elbows straight. With your hands still clasped, touch the toes on your right foot. Now stretch up to the starting position and drop down to the left foot, keeping your hands clasped. *(Figure 32)*

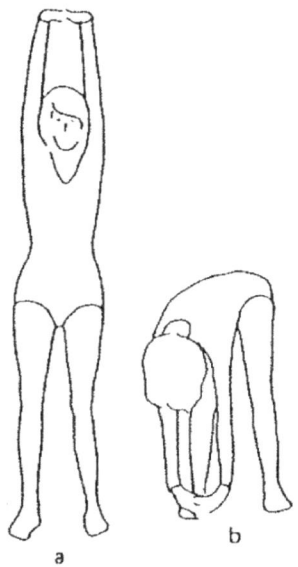

a   b

Figure 32

Limbo Stretch

Stand with your feet spread shoulder width apart and your hands on your hips. Lower yourself by bending your knees and tilting upper body backward (like a stiff board). Go as low and far back as you can with your face forward and upward--don't drop your head back. Remember to keep your feet flat on the floor. You should feel pull across your front from your chest to your thighs. *(Figure 33)*

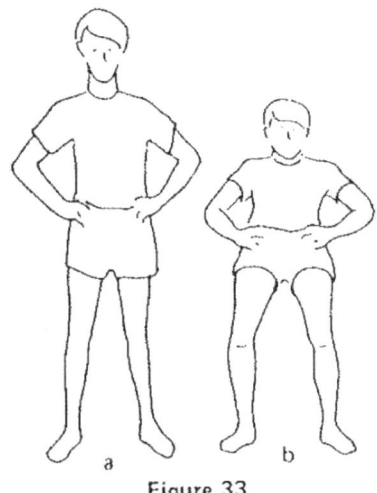

Figure 33

Limbo Bounce

Standing in the same position as in the Limbo Stretch, bend down and back as far as you can. Now bounce by lifting only your heels off the floor and then put them down again. Bounce several times and then bring yourself up to a straight standing position. Repeat.

Circle Stretch

Lower yourself by bending your knees and leaning back just as before in the Limbo Stretch and Limbo Bounce. Now lead with your hips; first to the left side, then to the back, then to the right side, and then back to the front. Keep your head in the same spot as your hips move in a circle. You should feel the pull particularly through the outside of your thighs. It's working! *(Figure 34)*

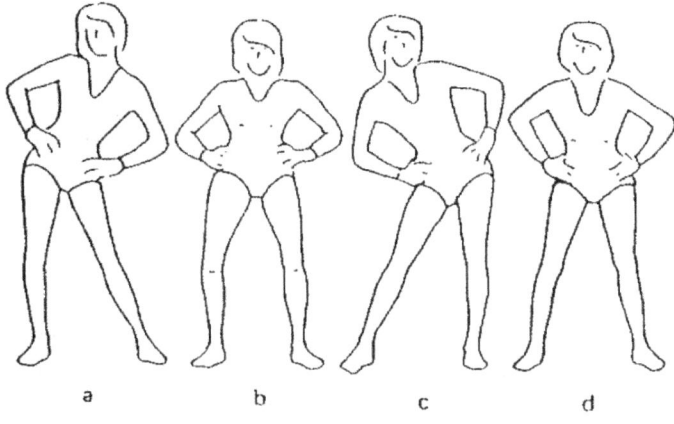

Figure 34

Thigh Stretcher

Standing with your feet far apart, move to the right side until your weight is over your right leg, keeping your right foot on the floor until you feel a stretch in the left thigh. The right knee should be bent and the left one should be straight. Hold--alternate sides and repeat. *(Figure 35)*

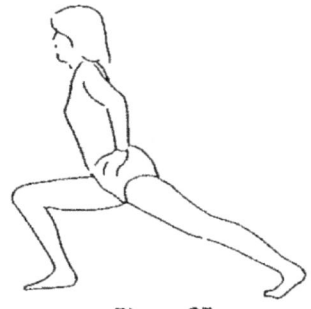

Figure 35

Head to Knees

Standing with your feet spread shoulder width apart and your knees straight, bend down until your forehead touches your knees. You may hold the back of your calves to help you. Now come up to a straight stand. Repeat. *(Figure 36)*

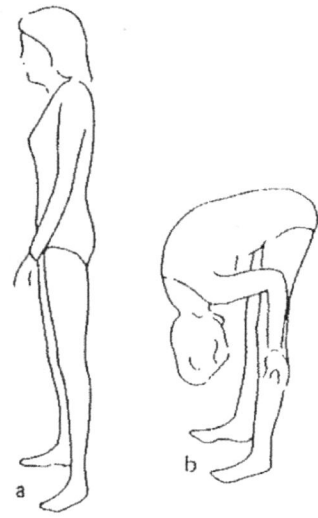

Figure 36

Sit on the floor with your legs stretched out in a "V." Keep your legs stretched as far as possible for the greatest results.

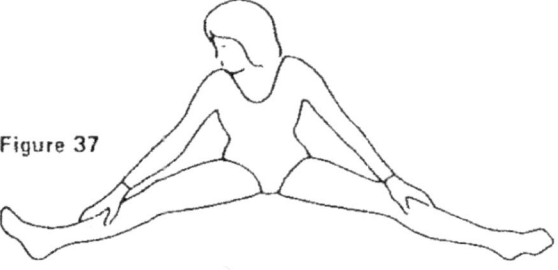

Figure 37

Hands to Toes

Sitting in this position, touch your right hand to your right foot, resting your left hand at your side. Then left hand to left foot. Repeat.

Both Hands to Both Feet

Keeping your legs as far apart as possible, touch both feet at the same time-- right hand to right foot, and left hand to left foot. *(Figure 38)*

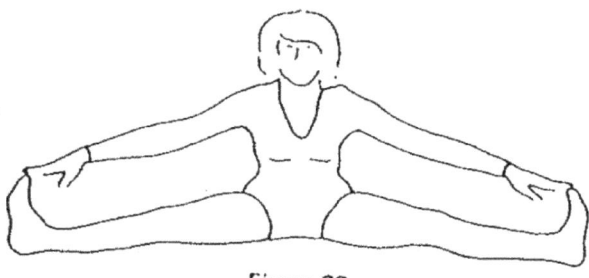

Figure 38

Toe to Toe Swing

With both arms together, and outstretched, point your fingers forward and touch first the right foot and then the left foot. Keep your hands in a straight line moving from side to side. Keep your body slightly forward.

Head to Knees

Sitting in the V-stretch position, put your forehead to your right knee. Alternate and put your forehead on your left knee. *(Figure 39)*.

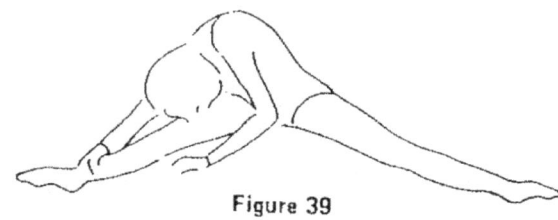

Figure 39

Hands Behind Neck/Elbow to Side

Clasp your hands behind your neck. Pull your elbows back as if trying to make a straight line from elbow to elbow. Touch the floor on the right side behind leg with right elbow. Then touch the floor on the left side behind leg with your right elbow. Alternate and touch floor on left side behind your leg with your left elbow and then touch the right side with the left elbow. *(Figure 40)*

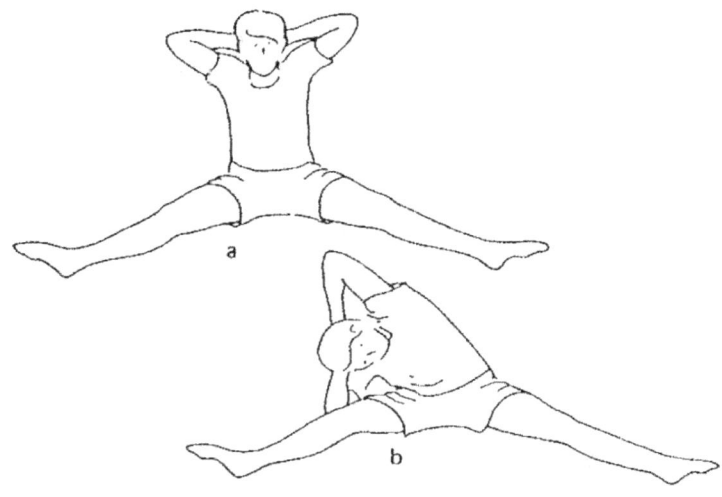

Figure 40

Hands Behind Neck/Elbows in Front

Clasp your hands behind your neck, bring your elbows forward. Then touch the floor between your legs with both elbows. Remember to keep your knees straight. *(Figure 41)*

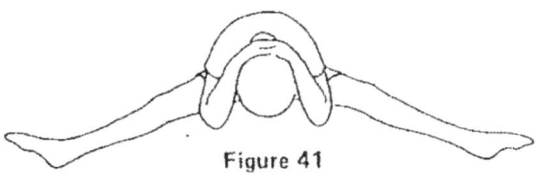

Figure 41

Clasp Hands Overhead--Touch Toes

Again, sitting in the V-position, clasp your hands and lace fingers. Hold your arms straight up overhead, keeping your elbows straight. Without relaxing your elbows, touch the right foot. Come up straight to sitting position, keeping elbows straight and lift your arms straight overhead. Then with clasped hands, touch the left foot and sit up straight again. Repeat. *(Figure 42)*

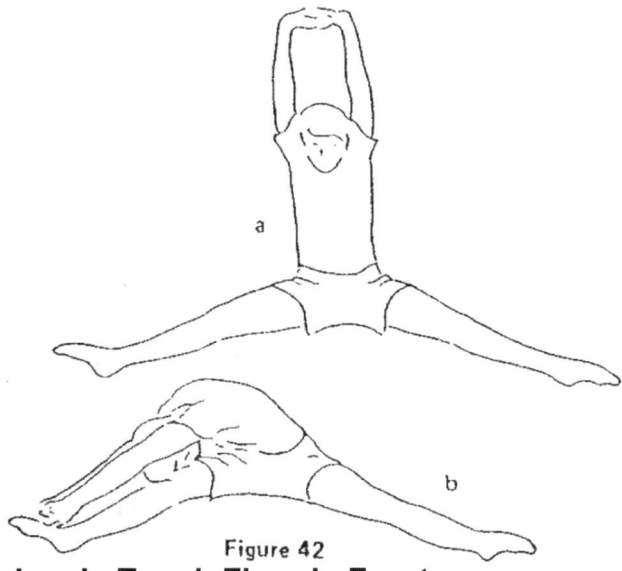

Figure 42

Clasp Hands Overhead - Touch Floor in Front

Clasp your hands overhead with your fingers laced and elbows straight. Lean forward and touch the floor in front of you. Your head should be near the floor. Then come up to a sitting position with your hands overhead again, still clasped and elbows straight. *(Figure 43)*

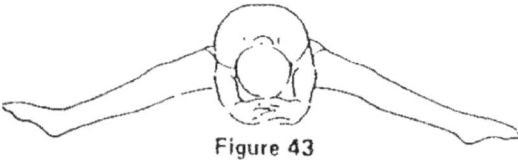

Figure 43

For the next exercises, sit with your legs stretched straight forward and your knees straight.

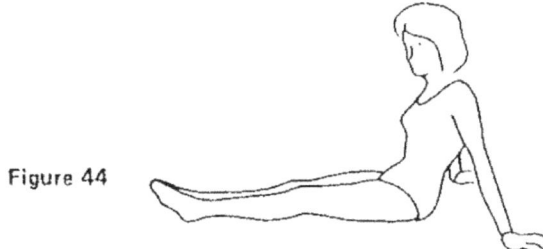

Figure 44

Lean Forward/Head to Knees

Sit with your legs outstretched and toes pointed forward. Then lean forward, moving your chest downward and your head to your knees. Let your arms move forward, keeping your knees straight. You'll feel pull in the legs, particularly behind the knees.

Lean Forward/Chest to Knees

Take hold of your feet, pull your chest down toward your knees. You may never get your chest down to your knees, but the harder you try the closer you'll get, and the greater benefits you'll have. *(Figure 45)*

35

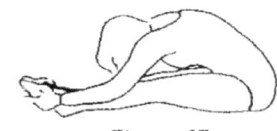

Figure 45

Hold Each Leg Up by Foot

Sit in V-stretch position again. Now hold both your feet from the inside, around the instep. First, raise your right leg straight up; then straighten your knee.

Note: If your knee does not straighten, try pressing on your right knee with your left hand. Do the same with the left leg.

Lift both legs up in the same manner, keeping your knees straight. Try to hold this position for a few moments. Almost everyone will find a balance spot if you lean back enough. If you find it, it will make the exercise easier. *(Figure 46)*

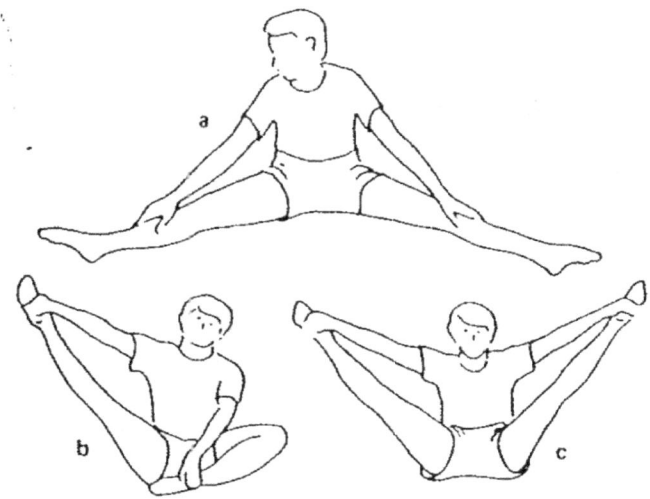

Figure 46

Raise Each Leg

For this exercise, lie on your left side. Support your head on your left hand, elbow on the floor. Raise right arm straight up from the shoulder. Raise right leg up to touch right hand. Lie on your right side and do the same with the left arm and leg. *(Figure 47)*

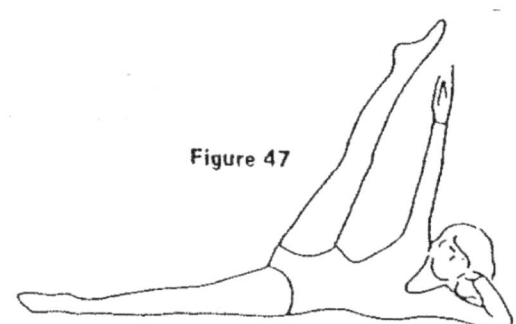

Figure 47

The next three exercises will be variations of the straight kneel position.

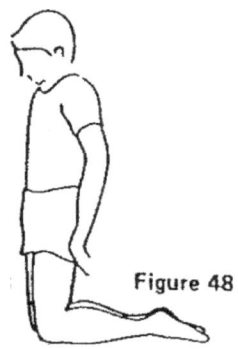

Figure 48

Rise to Side

Sitting with your hands on your ankles and your ankles by the sides of your legs, raise yourself up and out to the right, then lower yourself to a sitting position. Repeat. *(Figure 49)*

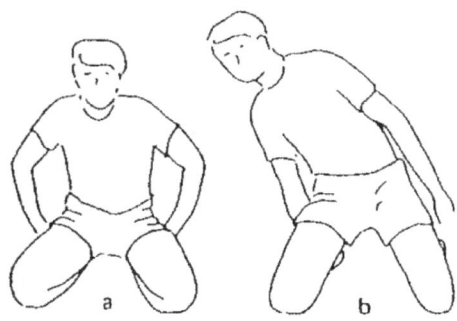

Figure 49

Fish

While still in a kneeling position, lean back and hold your feet or ankles. Now drop to your elbows; and come back up. *(Figure 50)*

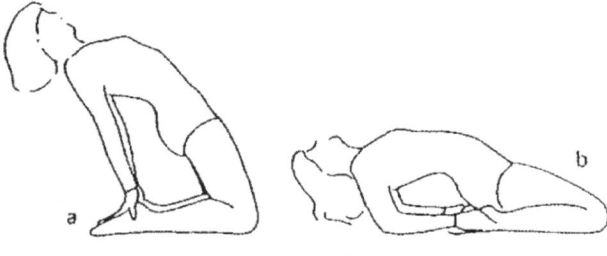

Figure 50

Look, Mom--No Hands!

Kneeling, extend arms straight in front of you. Now lean back until you are about four inches from the floor. Be sure to arch your back. Don't try to sit! Now come up to a straight kneel.

Do this exercise slowly. If you are afraid of hitting your head, use padding. *(Figure 51)*

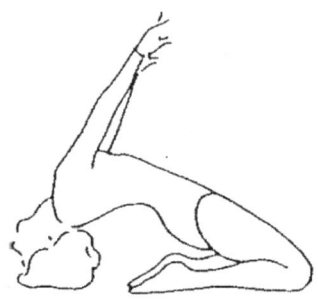

Figure 51

Weight Lifting

Use three-pound ladies' dumbbells or five-pound men's dumbbells. Or, if you're really ambitious, use dumbbells with interchangeable weights. Start with the lighter weights and add on.

Standing with one weight in each hand, touch the floor in front of your toes with the weights. Do not bend your knees. Then *stretch* up, reaching as high as possible. Repeat.

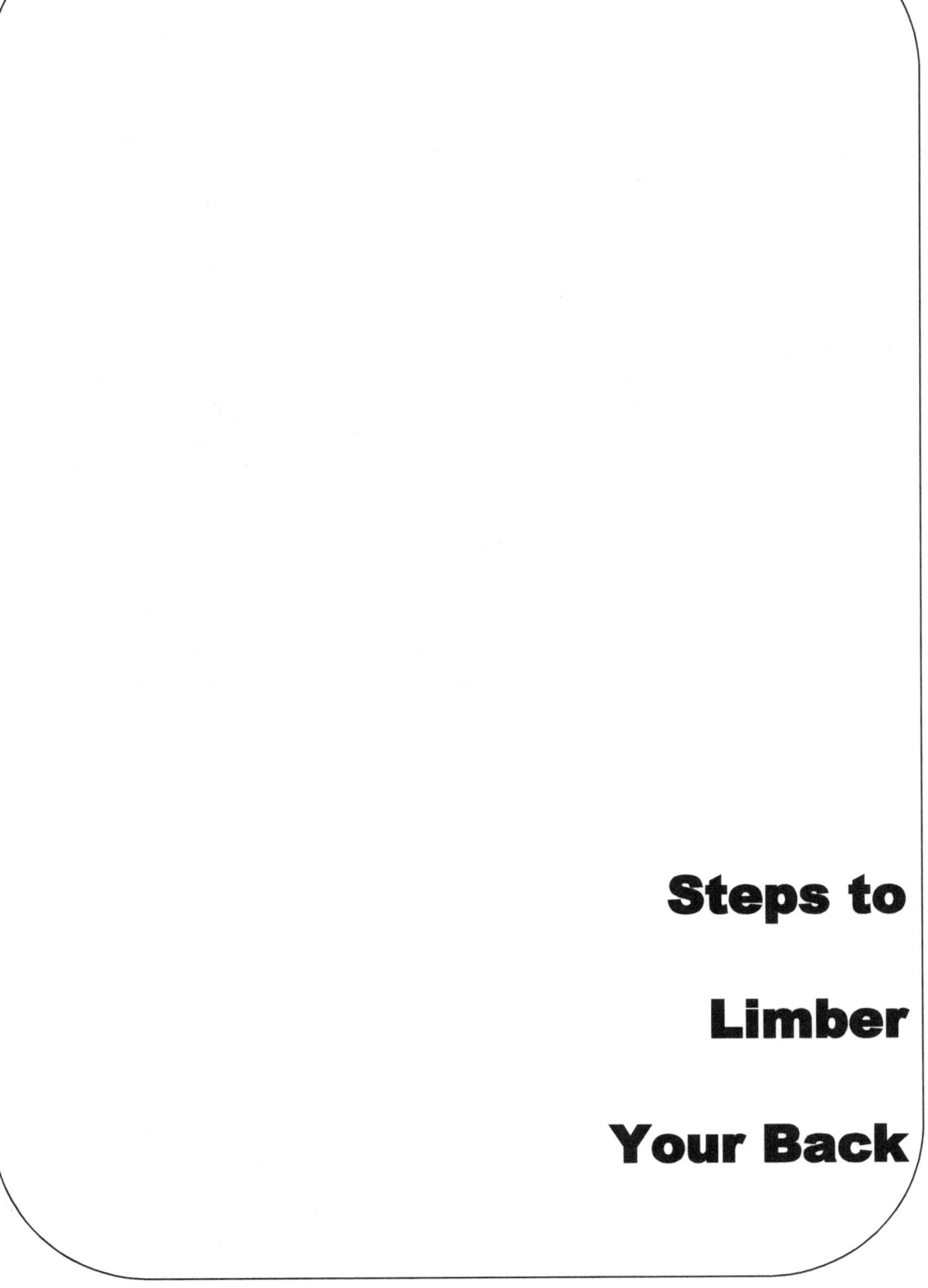

Steps to

Limber

Your Back

(Turn Your Back on Stiffness)

Spine to Floor

Lie on your back with legs extended. Push your spine (from the top to the bottom) flat down to the floor, keeping your heels and legs on the floor. Lift your hips upward, but do not lift the buttocks. Try to put your hands between your lower spine and the floor. If you are doing the exercise correctly, you should not be able to slide them under your back.

It may be impossible to get your spine all the way down to the floor with the first few tries, but it will get easier each time.

Body Stretch

Lie on your back with your legs extended and your arms above your head; palms up and elbows slightly bent. Stretch and pull your right arm up and at the same time pull down with the heel of your right foot. Stretch and pull several times. Now stretch up with your left arm and down with the heel of your left foot. Repeat. *(Figure 52)*

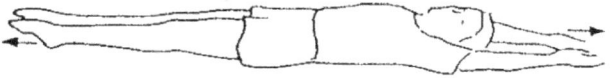

Figure 52

For the next five exercises, stand with your feet flat on the floor (except where otherwise indicated), feet spread shoulder width apart and knees straight. (Figure 53)

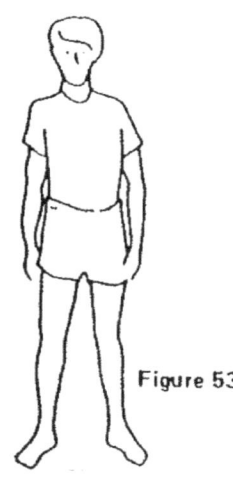

Figure 53

Regular Toe Touch

Standing, bend over and touch your toes with the tips of your fingers. Keep your knees and legs straight. Then, *stretch* up, reaching as high as possible. Repeat.

Toe Touch/Hands to Floor

Standing, bend over and touch the floor with the palms of your hands. Do not bend your knees. *Stretch* way up with arms, palms upward. Repeat.

Fan Toe Touch

Stand with your feet spread shoulder width apart and your arms outstretched. With your right hand, touch your left toes. Stand up and *stretch* with your arms up *high.* Then try your left hand to your right toes. Remember to keep your knees straight. Repeat. *(Figure 54)*

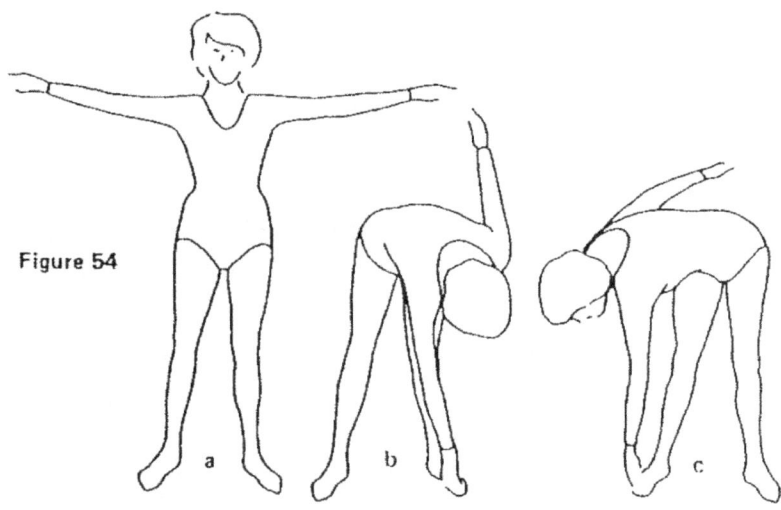

Figure 54

Knee Bend

Again, hold your arms straight out. Bend your knees and go down into a squatting position with your feet flat on floor. Then stand up straight. Repeat.

Knee Bend--Lift Heels Off Floor

Stand and hold your arms straight out. Bend your knees and go down into a squatting postion as before--with feet *flat on the floor.* Now lift your heels *high* up off the floor. Then put heels down again, still holding the squatting position with your arms outstretched. Stand up and repeat.

Half Sit Ups

With legs and knees straight, lie back with arms outstretched. Sit up as far as you can, with your lower back still on the floor. Repeat. Smile--you're toning up! *(Figure 55)*

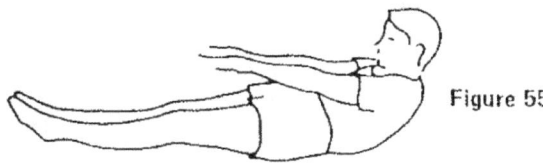

Figure 55

Back Over

Lie on your back. Now bring hips up and support them with your hands. Try to straighten legs back up and over your head and then touch toes to the ground way above your head. Repeat. *(Figure 56)*

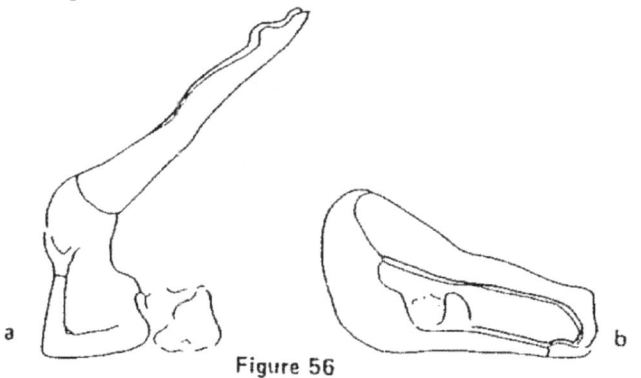

Figure 56

Roll Up to Shoulders

Lying on your back, bring your knees up to your buttocks. Hold your ankles to either side and *slowly* roll up inch-by-inch from the buttocks, until you are high up on your shoulders. Now come down slowly, bringing lower back down before buttocks. *(Figure 57)*

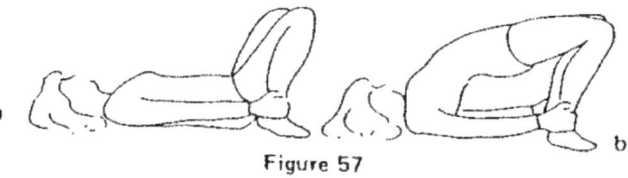

Figure 57

Spine Rock

Sit with your knees up and bent, and your feet crossed. Grasp your feet with your hands. Then rock back onto your shoulders. Rock from side to side and come back into a sitting position, pushing off from the floor with your middle back. Remember to keep your feet in a crossed position. *(Figure 58)*

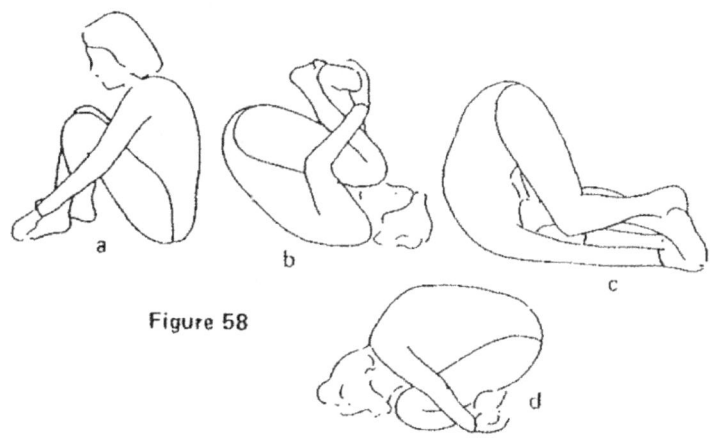

Figure 58

Plough

Lie on your back with arms stretched straight up overhead. Lift your legs up all the way past your head and take hold of your feet with your hands. Now move feet apart and together (about 6 inches). *(Figure 59)*

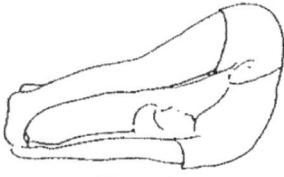

Figure 59

Shoulder Balance

Roll up onto shoulders. Bring your legs straight up. Do not bend your knees. Now bring your hands up alongside your legs and balance for a few moments. *(Figure 60)*

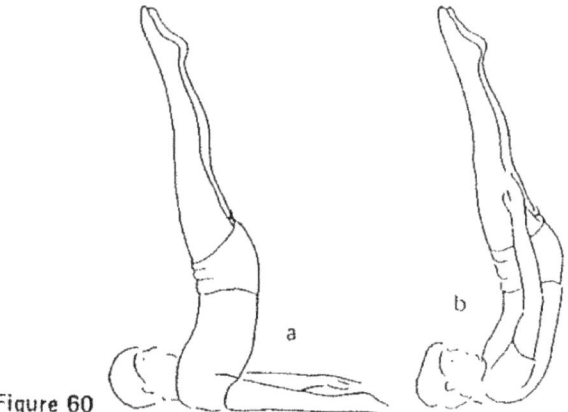

Figure 60

For the next two exercises, get down on all fours. Place palms shoulder width apart and fingers slightly to the side. (Figure 61)

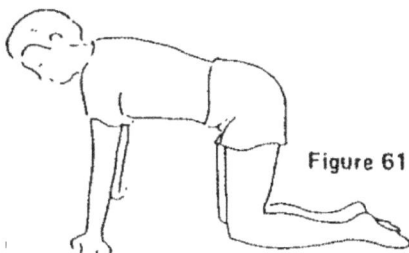

Figure 61

Back Pick Up and Drop

Raise your back as high and rounded as you can. Now push out your lower back to get it as low and arched as you can. Repeat.

Knees to Elbow

Again, on all fours, bring your right knee up to your right elbow. Repeat this three times. Now do the same with the left knee. Repeat the whole exercise. *(Figure 62)*

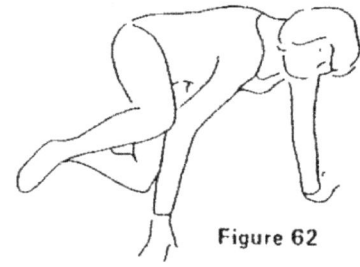

Figure 62

Sit Down On Feet/Arch Back

Kneel straight up. Arch back, stomach and chest out. Lower yourself, until you are sitting on your feet. With your back still arched, rise up to a straight kneel. *(Figure 63)*

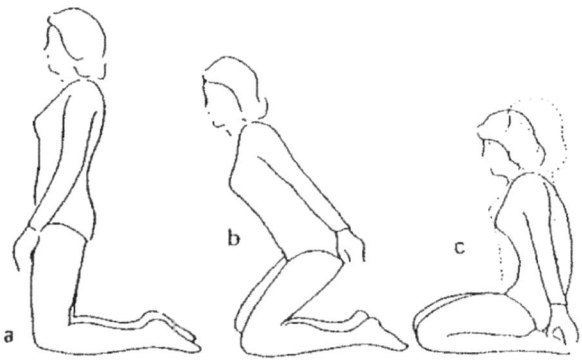

Figure 63

Sit Back On Calves/Chest to Knees

Kneeling with your back straight, lower yourself until you are sitting on your feet. Now bend forward and put chest to knees. Keep your back straight and come up to a straight kneel. *(Figure 64)*

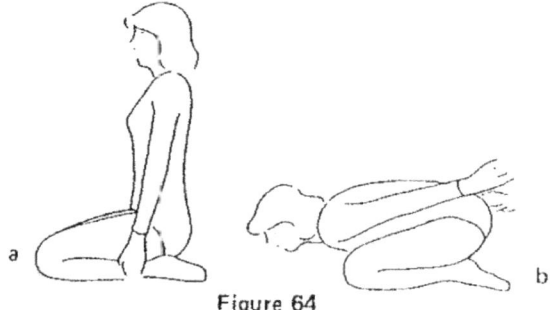

Figure 64

Weight Lifting

Use three-pound ladies' dumbbells or five-pound men's dumbbells. Or, if you're really ambitious, use dumbbells with interchangeable weights. Start with the lighter weights and add on.

Half Sit Ups

With one weight in each hand, lie back with your arms stretched straight above your head. Sit up as far as you can with your lower back still on the floor and lift your arms as far as possible. *(Figure 65)*

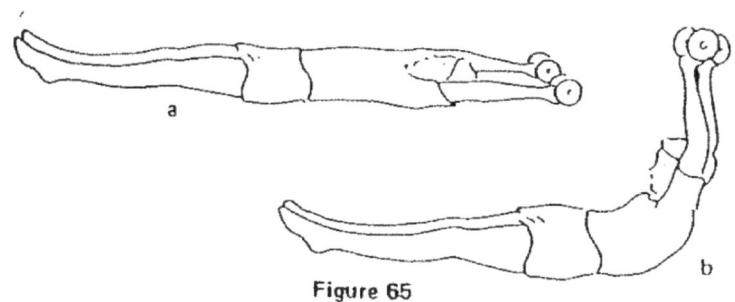

Figure 65

Sit Ups

With one weight in each hand, lie back with your arms stretched overhead. Sit up and touch about an inch in front of your toes with the weights. Be careful not to drop the weights on your feet. Keep your knees straight and your heels on the floor. It will be easier to keep your feet on the floor if you point your toes. *(Figure 66)*

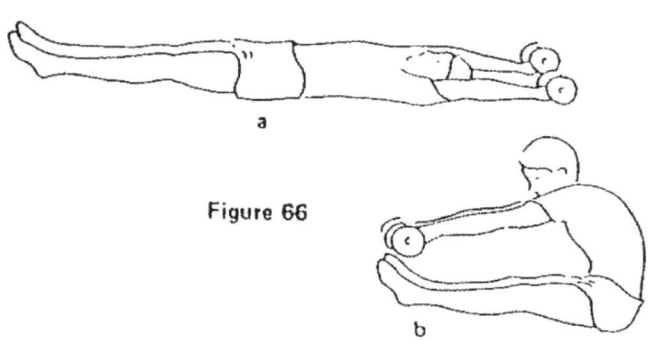

Figure 66

Toe Touch

Standing with one weight in each hand, touch the floor in front of your toes with the weights. Keep your knees straight. *Stretch* up, reaching as high as possible. Repeat. *(Figure 67)*

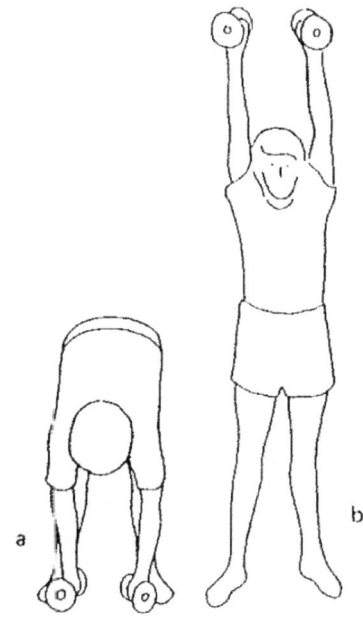

a   b

Figure 67

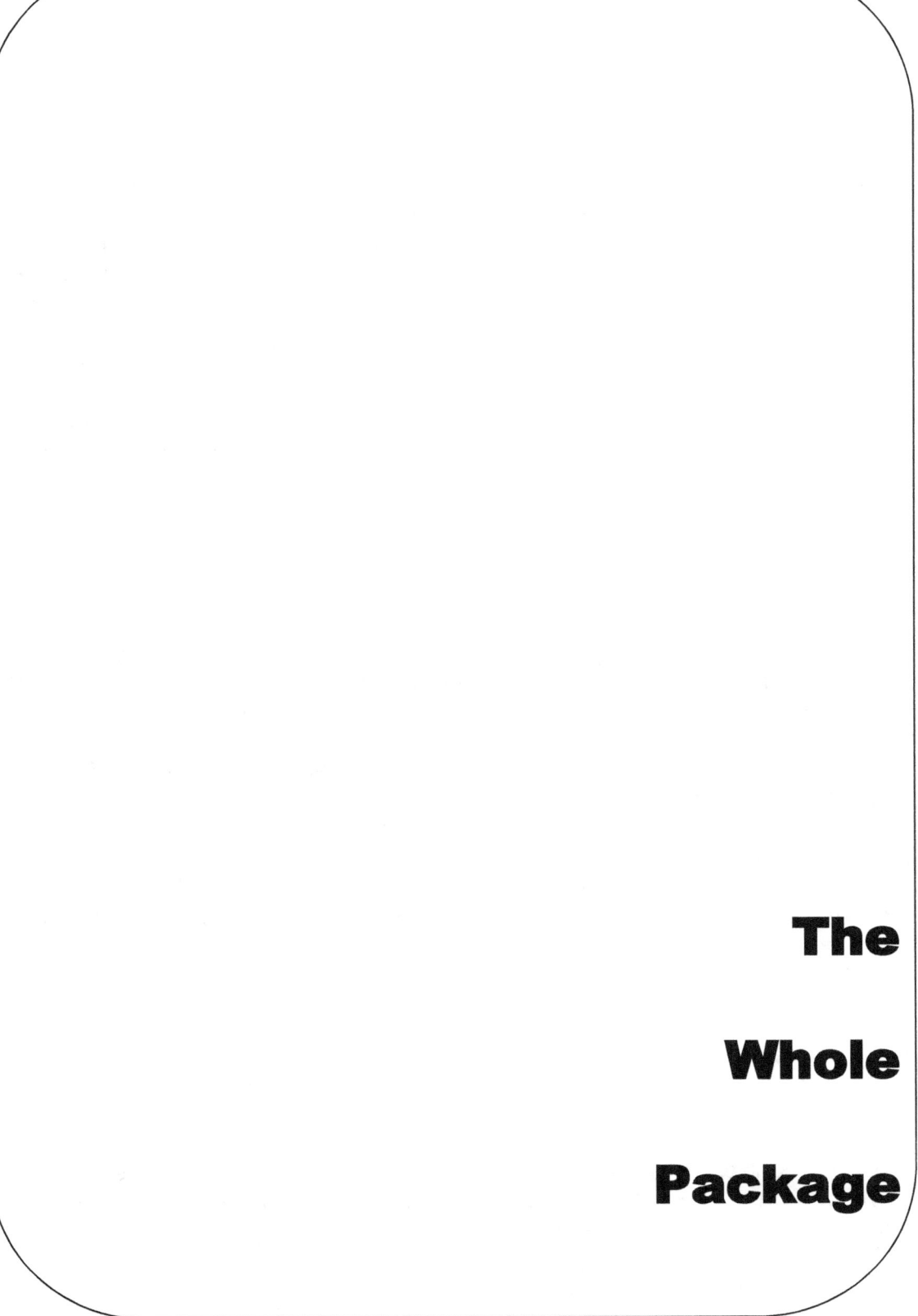

The

Whole

Package

(A Healthy Sampling for the Whole System....)

Spine to Floor

Lie on your back with your legs extended. Push your spine (from the top to the bottom) flat down to the floor; keeping your heels and legs on the floor. Lift your hips, but not the buttocks. Try to put your hands between your lower spine and the floor. If you *cannot* get them between, you are doing this exercise correctly.

It may be impossible to get your spine all the way down to the floor with the first few tries, but it will get easier each time.

This exercise is particularly good for people with lower back problems. Starting the exercise program with this stretcher will help in the following exercises.

Most beneficial to : Lower back.

Neck to Floor

Lie on your back with your legs extended. Push the back of your neck flat down to the floor. Do this by pulling your chin down toward your chest; but don't lift your head off the floor. When you are doing this one correctly, you will not be able to get your fingers underneath your neck.

This exercise does not come easy to everyone. However, after a few sessions, you should be able to do it.

Spine and Neck to Floor at Same Time

Lying on your back with your leg extended, push both spine and neck to the floor just as before, but at *the same time.* You will feel even more stretch with exercise. *(Figure 68)*

Most beneficial to : Both back and nec.k

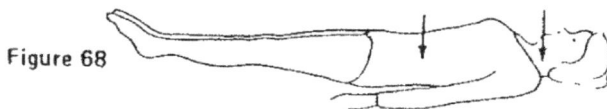

Figure 68

Body Stretch

Lie on your back with your legs straight out and your arms above your head: palms up and elbows slightly bent. Stretch and pull your right arm up and at the same time pull down with the heel of your right foot. Repeat.

You should feel pull in the upper arms and your calves.

Most beneficial to: Back, arms, and legs.

Overhead Stretch

Sit down on the floor with your legs crossed. Keep your back straight. First with your right hand reach way, way up, as far as you can reach. Then do the same on the left side.

You will feel pull through the middle. If you cannot feel the pull, stretch a little harder. *(Figure 69)*

Most beneficial to: Waist.

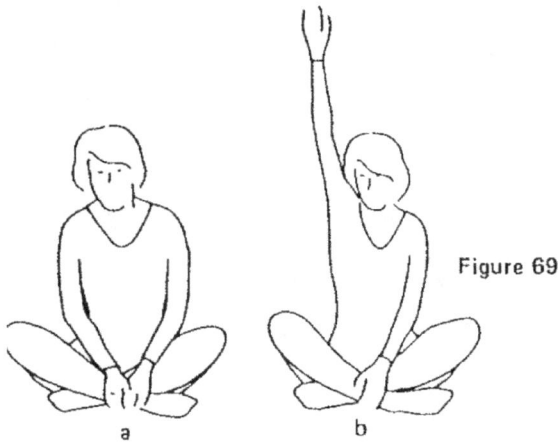

Figure 69

Overhead Stretch/Wrist

Sitting on the floor and with your legs crossed, stretch up with your right arm. With left hand, take hold of your right wrist and pull down while leaning slightly to the left. Now stretch up with the left arm. With right hand, take hold of your left wrist and pull while leaning slightly to the right.

Again, you will feel pull in the side waist area, and also the arms. *(Figure 70)*

Most beneficial to: Waist and arms.

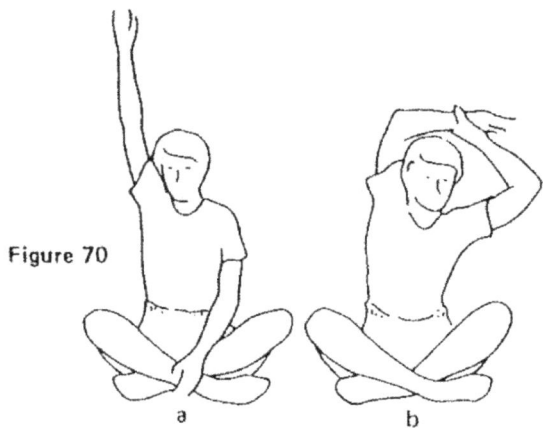

Figure 70

Overhead Side Stretch

While sitting in the same position, keeping your body straight, stretch up and over your head with your right arm. Then do the same with your left arm. This is another great one for both the waist and arms. *(Figure 71)*

Most beneficial to: Waist.

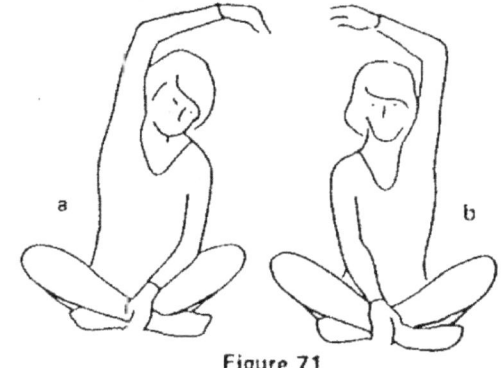

Figure 71

Head to Floor

Sit cross-legged and bend from your lower back forward, touching your head to the floor in front of your feet.

This is not only a great stretcher for the lower back, but your thighs will feel it, too. *(Figure 72)*

Most beneficial to: Legs and back.

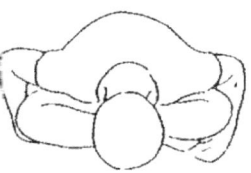

Figure 72

Before starting these next exercises, let's warm up by sitting with the soles of your feet together. Now take hold of your feet with your hands. Bring your heels toward you and lean forward at the same time. As you are doing this, try to pull your knees downward without using your hands. Repeat.

The next four exercises are basically the same as we have just completed, but they are done with the soles of your feet together. This will give the same pulls as before with a little extra pull through the thighs. (Figure 73)

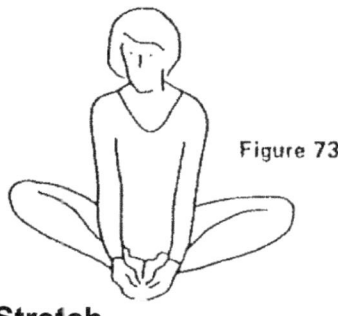

Figure 73

Soles Together Overhead Stretch

With your right hand, stretch upward while keeping your left hand on your left knee, stretch as high as you can. Now do the same with the left hand, putting your right hand on your right knee.

Most beneficial to: Thighs and waist.

Soles Together Overhead Stretch/Wrist

Stretch up with your right arm. With the left hand, grab your right wrist and pull down toward your head, while slightly leaning to the left. Then alternate sides--stretch up with your left arm, right hand grabs left wrist and pull while leaning slightly to the right. Repeat.

Most beneficial to: Thighs, waist and arms

Soles Together Overhead Side Stretch

Reach up and over your head with right arm. You may rest your left hand on your feet. Lean to the left just enough to feel a slight pull. Now do the same with the left hand up and over your head with the right hand on your feet. Repeat.

Most beneficial to: Thighs and waist.

Soles Together Head to Feet

Hold your feet with both hands. Bend forward and *stretch* until your head touches your feet. Do not lift your buttocks from the floor.

This one is hard to do at first, but each time it gets easier. This is a good one to repeat at the end of your session or workout. *(Figure 74)*

Most beneficial to: Thighs and back.

Figure 74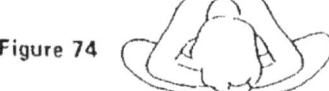

The next 24 exercises should be done standing, with your feet flat on the floor (except where otherwise indicated); feet spread shoulder width apart and knees straight. You should feel pulls through the side, waist and arms.

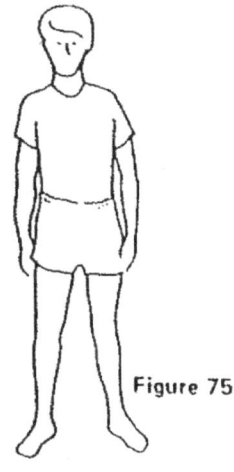

Figure 75

51

Standing Overhead Stretch

Stretch your right arms up high above your head, reaching with your fingertips as high as you can. Then stretch your left arm up the same way. Repeat.
Most beneficial to: Waist.

Standing Overhead Stretch/Wrist

Stretch up with your right arm. With your left hand, grab the right wrist and pull down over your head while slightly leaning to the left. Stretch upward with the left arm. With the right hand, grab the left wrist and pull down while leaning slightly to the right. Repeat, alternating sides.
Most beneficial to: Waist and arms.

Standing Overhead Side Stretch

Stretch up and over your head with your right arm and lean slightly to the left. Now stretch over your head with the left arm, while leaning slightly to the right.
Most beneficial to: Waist.

These next six exercises will pull on your legs and thighs, as well as stretch the lower back.

Standing Toe Touch

Touch your toes with the tips of your fingers, keeping your legs straight. *Stretch* up, reaching as high as possible. Repeat. *(Figure 76)*
Most beneficial to: Legs, back and stomach.

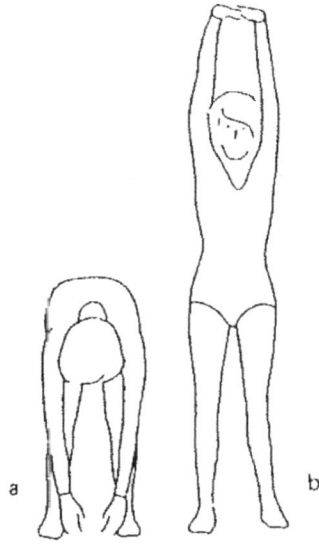

Figure 76

Standing Rag Doll Flop

Touch the floor in front of your toes with the tips of your fingers. Come up about six inches off the floor and then down again. Repeat eight times. Then reach with hands *high* up over your head and repeat. Do not bend your knees! *(Figure 77)*

Most beneficial to: Legs, back and stomach

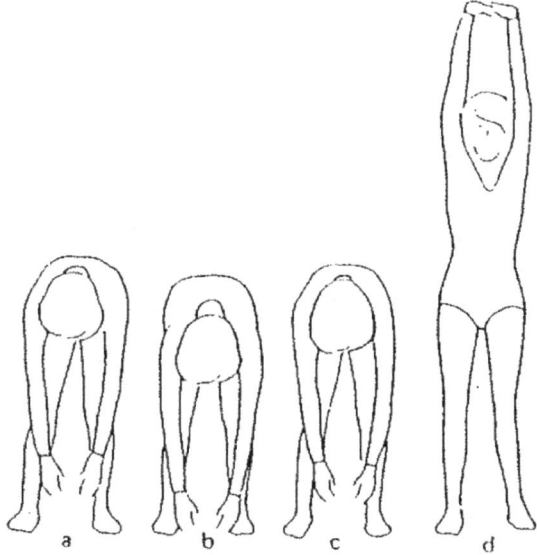

Figure 77

Standing Fan Toe Touch
Stand with your feet spread shoulder width apart and arms outstretched. Now with your right hand, touch your left toes with the tips of your fingers. Come up and *stretch* with your arms up *high.* Then left hand to the right toes. Again, do not bend knees. Repeat.

Most beneficial to: Legs, back and stomach.

Standing Toe Touch/Clasped Hands
With your feet spread shoulder width apart and standing with clasped hands and fingers laced; lift arms overhead, with elbows straight. Keeping your hands clasped, touch the toes on your right foot. Now stretch up to the starting positon, then down to the left foot, with your hands still clasped. (Figure 78)

Most beneficial to: Legs, back, stomach and arms.

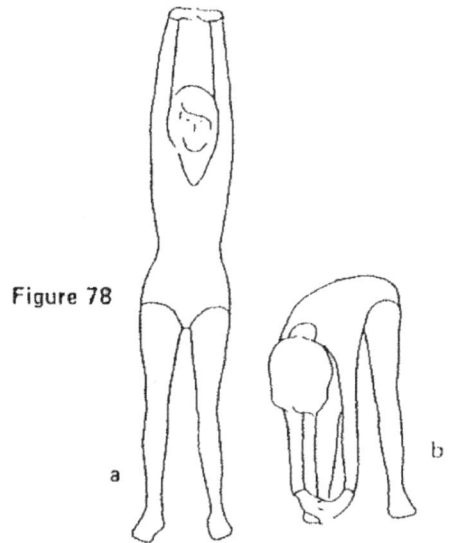

Figure 78

a

b

Standing Toe Touch/Crossed Legs

Standing erect, cross your legs with feet shoulder width apart. Now touch your toes (right hand touches left foot, and left hand touches right foot). Hold for a few seconds. Come up to a straight stand and stretch arms way up. Repeat. *(Figure 79)*

Most beneficial to: Legs, back, stomach and arms.

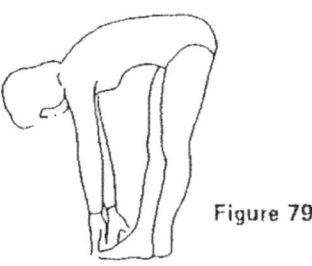

Figure 79

Standing Limbo Stretch

Stand, with feet shoulder width apart and hands on hips. Lower yourself by bending your knees and tilting upper body backward (like a stiff board). Go as low and far back as you can. Keep your face forward and upward--don't drop your head back. Keep your feet flat on the floor. Smile! You should feel pull from your chest to your thighs. *(Figure 80)*

Most beneficial to: Legs, stomach and back.

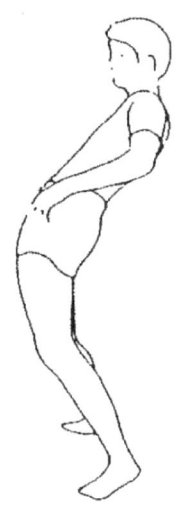

Figure 80

Standing Limbo Bounce

Again, the same position as in the Limbo Stretch (feet spread shoulder width apart and hands on hips). Bend down and back as far as you can. Now bounce by lifting only your heels off the floor and then put them down again. Bounce several times and then bring yourself up to a straight standing position. Repeat.

Again, you will feel this pull across your front from your chest to your thighs.

Most beneficial to: Legs, stomach and back.

Standing Circle Stretch

Lower yourself by bending your knees and leaning back just as before in the Limbo Stretch and Limbo Bounce. Now lead with your hips, first to the left side, then to the back, then to the right side, and then back to the front. Your head should stay in the same spot as you are going around the circle with your hips.

The pull should feel particularly strong through the outside of your thighs. *(Figure 81)*. Smile--it's working!

Most beneficial to: Legs, stomach and back.

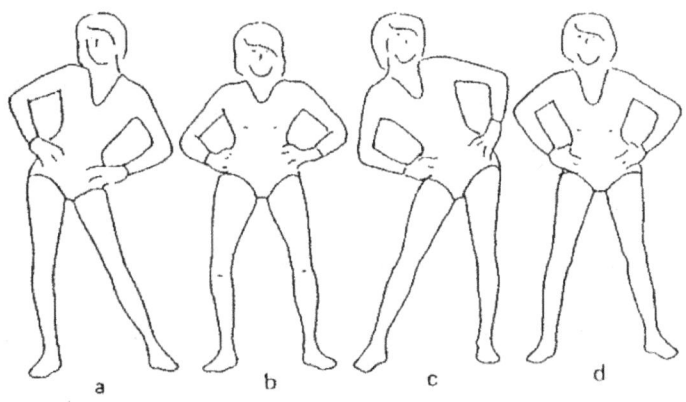

Figure 81

Circle Bounce

Start the same way as the Circle Stretch, but bounce once in each direction (front, left, back, right). Bounce by lifting your heels only off the floor and down again. Then try this with *two* bounces in each direction.

You'll feel pull across the front.

Most beneficial to: Legs, stomach and back.

Wrist Circles

Stand straight with your feet spread shoulder width apart. Extend your arms from your sides at shoulder height, palms up. Make small circles forward with hands. Now make small circles backwards with your palms down.

Most beneficial to: Arms and wrists.

Half Knee Bends

Extend your arms straight forward, palms down. Bend knees halfway. For most of us that point is a "Shakey" one. Then stand up straight. Do this exercise very slowly. Remember---feet flat on the floor.

This is good for your legs and for balance. *(Figure 82)*

Most beneficial to: Legs and lower back.

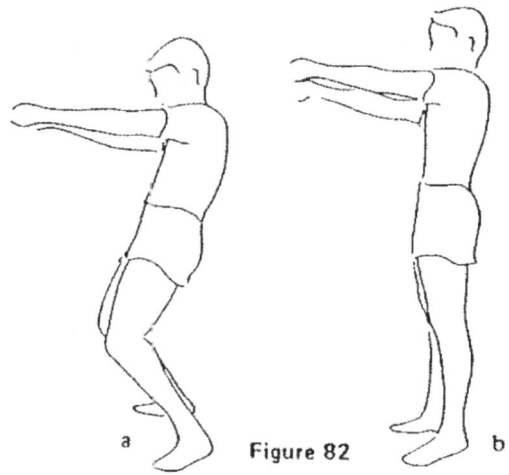

a   Figure 82   b

Knee Bend

Hold your arms straight out. Bend your knees and go down into a squatting position with feet flat on floor. Then stand up straight. Repeat.

Most beneficial to: Legs and lower back.

Knee Bend--Heel Lift

Hold your arms straight out. Bend your knees and go down into a squatting position as before--with feet flat on the floor. Now lift your heels high up off the floor. Then put your heels down again, still being in the squatting position with arms outstretched. Now stand up. Repeat.

Most beneficial to: Legs and lower back.

Thigh Stretcher

Standing with your feet far apart, move to the right side until your weight is over your right leg, keeping feet flat on the floor until your feel a stretch in the left thigh. Right knee should be bent and left one should be straight. Alternate sides and repeat. Congratulations--you look better already! *(Figure 83)*

Most beneficial to: Thighs.

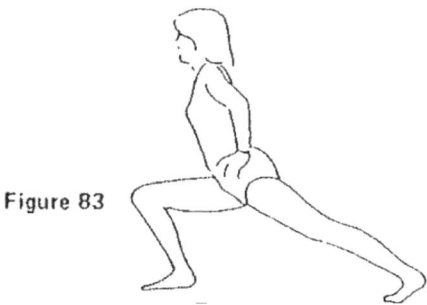
Figure 83

Knee Lift

Stand erect, feet together. Raise your right leg as high as possible, holding the front of your calf with your hands and pulling your knee against your body. Left foot must be flat on the floor and your back must be kept straight. Alternate sides.

Most beneficial to: Thighs, legs and lower back.

Shoulder Pull

With your right hand, reach over the right shoulder with your elbow pointing straight up; bring left hand behind back and grasp right hand, then pull. Now with left hand, reach over left shoulder with elbow pointing straight up; then bring right hand behind back and grasp left hand; pull. *(Figure 84)*

Most beneficial to: Back, stomach and arms.

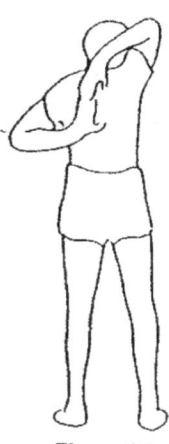
Figure 84

One Leg Stand

Stand erect. Then grab your left ankle with your right hand behind you. Stretch. Hold your body straight while balancing on one foot. Switch sides. This is another good balancing stretcher. *(Figure 85)*

Most beneficial to: Legs and balance.

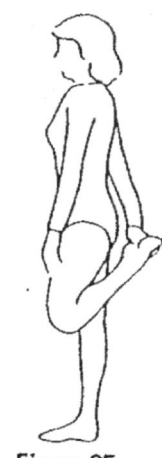

Figure 85

Body Bender

Standing straight, clasp your hands behind your neck with fingers laced. Pull your elbows back as if to make a straight line from elbow to elbow. Lean to the right side with your elbow as far as you can, keeping the rest of your body straight. Now do the same to the left side. *(Figure 86)*

Most beneficial to: Stomach, chest and sides.

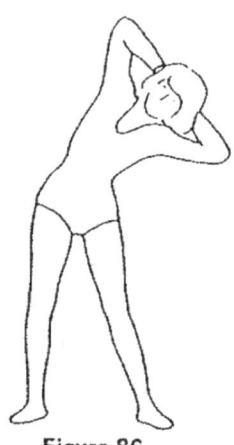

Figure 86

Head to Knees

Still standing with your feet spread shoulder width apart and knees straight, bend over until your forehead touches your knees. You may hold the back of your claves to help. Now come up to a straight stand. Repeat.

Most beneficial to: Legs and thighs.

Squat

Now get in a squatting position. Come up on the balls of your feet, keeping hands flat on the floor and fingers pointing toward each other. Roll forward, putting weight on your arms; dropping head forward and pushing chest against thighs. Roll forward and back and repeat. *(Figure 87)*

Most beneficial to: Legs.

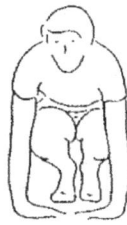

Figure 87

The next nine exercises will be done sitting with your legs stretched out in a "V." Keep your legs stretched as far apart as possible for the best results.

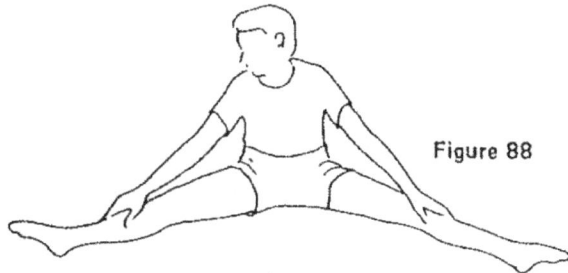

Figure 88

Hands to Toes

Sitting in this position, touch your right hand to your right foot, left hand resting at your side. Then left hand to left foot. Repeat.

Most beneficial to: Thighs

Both Hands to Both Feet

Keeping legs as far apart as possible, touch both your feet at the same time (right hand to right foot, and left hand to left foot). *(Figure 89)*

Most beneficial to; Thighs.

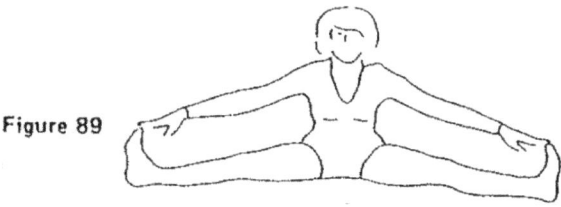

Figure 89

Toe to Toe Swing

With arms outstretched, and together, point fingers forward and swing hands from right foot to left foot. Keep hands in a straight line as you're swinging from foot to foot; and keep body forward.

Most beneficial to: Thighs.

Toe to Toe Swirl

Starting with both hands on your right foot, head pointed toward the right foot, move both hands to the left foot and reach over your head with your right arm. Hold your left ankle with your left hand and stretch from the waist around as far to the right as you can. Then turn back around to the front, bringing your right arm down to the left foot, and swing both hands back to the right foot. Reach over head around your face with your left arm. Turn head to the left, stretch from the waist around as far to the left as you can. Then turn back around to the front *(Figure 90)*

Most beneficial to: Thighs, stomach and back.

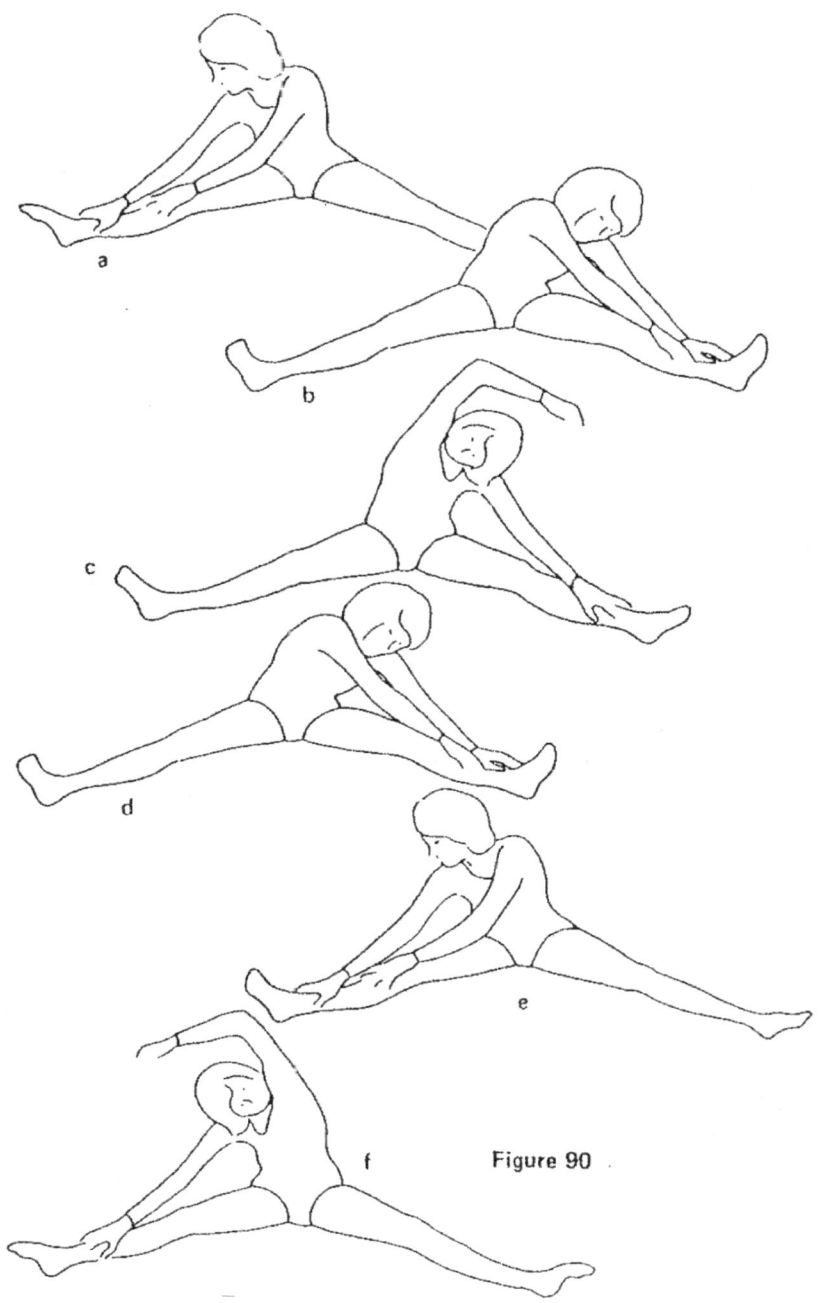

Figure 90

Head to Knees

Sitting in the V-stretch position, put your forehead to your right knee. Alternate and put your forehead on your left knee.

Most beneficial to: Thighs and back.

Hands Behind Neck/Elbow to Side

Clasp your hands behind your neck. Pull your elbows back as if trying to make a straight line between elbows. Touch the floor on the right side behind your leg with your right elbow. Then touch the floor on the left side behind your leg with your left elbow.

Most beneficial to: Thighs and stomach.

Hands Behind Neck/Elbows in Front

Clasp your hands behind your neck, bringing your elbows forward. Touch the floor between your legs with both elbows. Keep your knees straight. This one really works for you! *(Figure 91)*

Most beneficial to: Thighs and back.

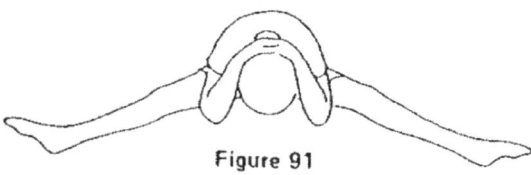

Figure 91

Clasp Hands Overhead--Touch Toes

Clasp your hands with laced fingers. Hold your arms overhead, with your elbows straight. Without relaxing your elbows, touch the right foot with hands clasped. Come up straight to a sitting position, keeping your elbows straight and lift your arms straight overhead. Then, with clasped hands, touch the left foot and sit straight up again. Repeat.

Most beneficial to: Thighs, back and arms.

Clasp Hands Overhead--Touch Floor in Front

Clasping your hands overhead with your fingers laced and elbows straight; touch the floor in front of you. Put your head down toward the floor. Keep your hands clasped and your arms straight. Come up to a sitting position with your hands overhead. Repeat. *(Figure 92)*

Most beneficial to: Thighs, arms and back.

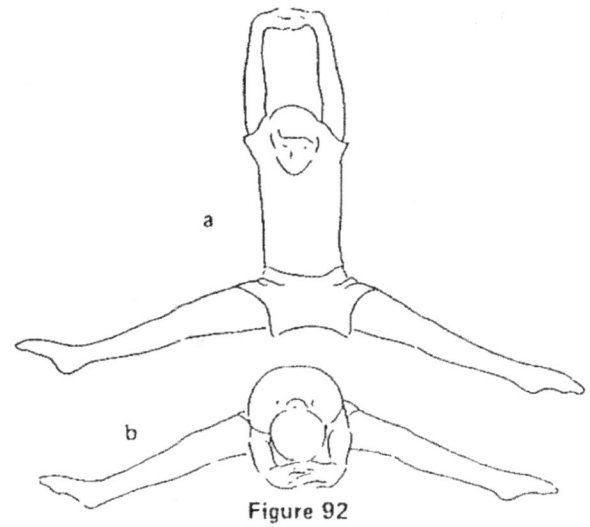

Figure 92

Exercises in the "V-stretch" position are excellent thigh stretchers.

V-Turn Pivot

Sitting in the V-stretch position, bring your right foot toward you, and your left foot to the left side. Turn around to your right, bringing your left arm with you and turning your right shoulder until you see your left foot. Turn back around, switch your legs so your left foot is toward you and your right foot is to the outside. Now bring your right arm with you and turn the left shoulder until you see your right foot. *(Figure 93)*

Most beneficial to: Thighs, stomach and back.

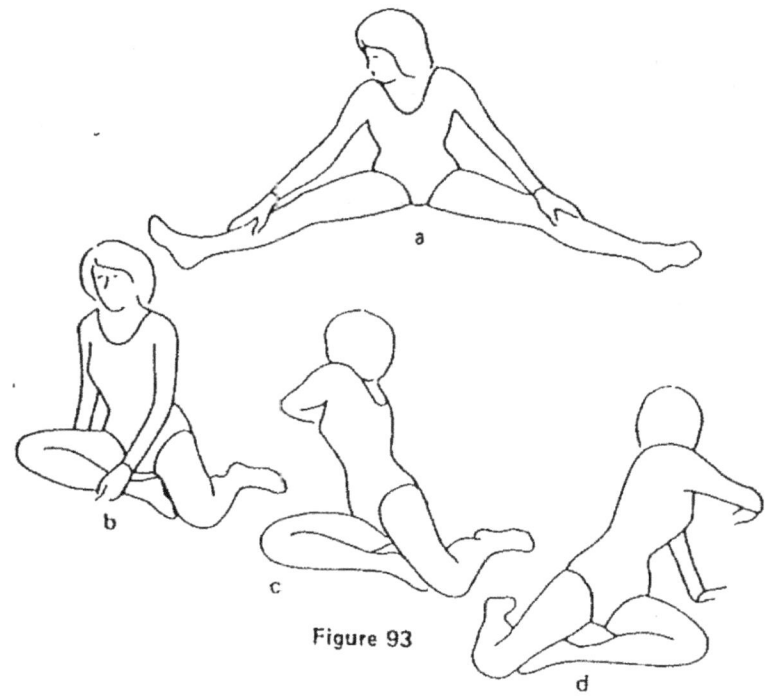

Figure 93

For the next ten exercises, you should sit with your legs stretched straight forward and your knees straight.

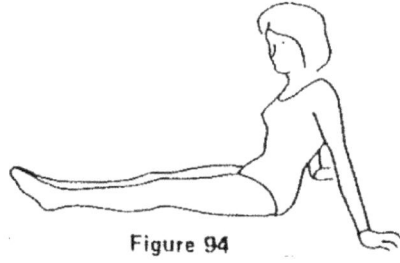

Figure 94

Exercise Feet

Bending from the ankles, move your feet forward, toes pointing away; and then back, toes pointing toward you. Then turn feet in circles. Now reverse the circles. *(Figure 95)*

Most beneficial to: Feet.

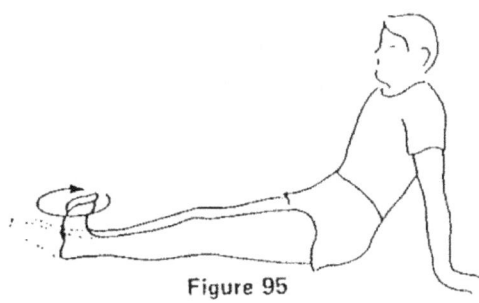

Figure 95

Lean Forward/Head to Knees

Sit with your legs outstretched and toes pointed. Lean forward, moving your chest downward and your head to your knees. Let your arms move forward. Do not bend knees.

You'll feel pull in the legs, particularly behind the knees.

Most beneficial to: Legs and back.

Lean Forward/Chest to Knees

Hold your toes and pull your chest down toward your knees. The harder you try, the closer you'll get, and the greater the benefits! *(Figure 96)*

Most beneficial to: Legs and back.

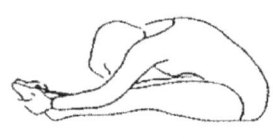

Figure 96

Curl Up

Lying flat on your back with your arms stretched overhead, bend the left knee with the sole flat on the floor. Raise your right leg straight up. Straighten knee.

Press waist to the floor. Curl forward while clasping hands behind knee. Alternate and repeat. *(Figure 97)*

Most beneficial to: Stomach and legs.

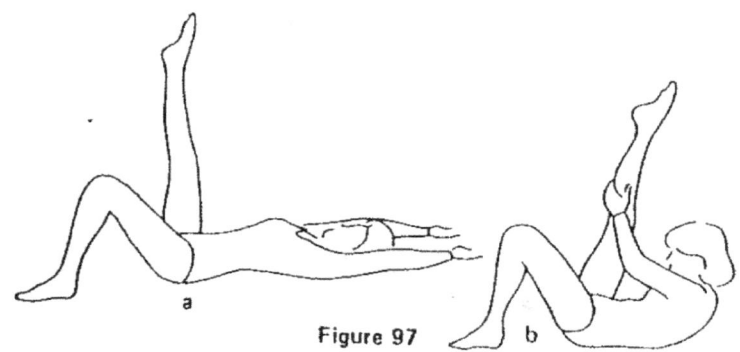

Figure 97

Inch Back

With your arms stretched forward on top of your legs, go back inch by inch, slowly, until your lower back is almost touching the floor, but not quite. Then sit up. Do this several times. Then go all the way back and stretch your arms straight overhead. Repeat. *(Figure 98)*

Most beneficial to: Stomach and back.

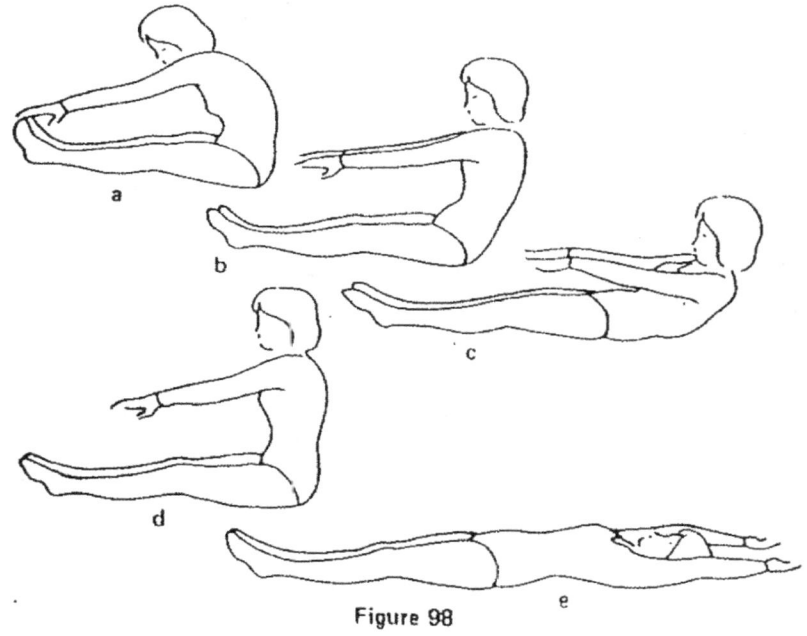

Figure 98

Sit Ups

Lie back with hands stretched straight overhead. Sit up and touch your toes with your hands. Keep your knees straight and your heels on the floor.

Most beneficial to: Stomach and back.

It will be easier to keep your feet on the floor if you point your toes forward!

Fan Sit Ups

Lie back with your hands stretched straight overhead. Sit up and touch the toes on the left foot with your right hand, and lie back again. Come up and touch the toes on the right foot with your left hand. Repeat.

Most beneficial to: Stomach, back and arms.

Half Sit Ups

Lie back with your arms outstretched. Sit up as far as you can with your lower back still on the floor. Repeat. *(Figure 99)*

Most beneficial to: Back and stomach.

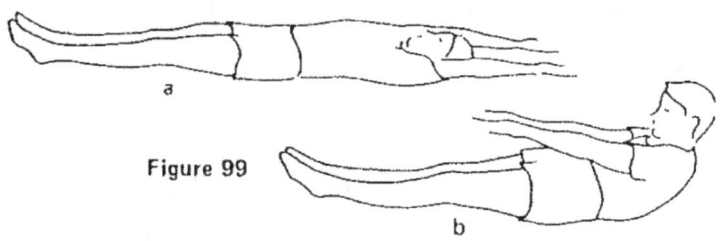

Figure 99

Back Over

Lie on your back. Bring your hips up and support them with your hands. Straighten your legs back up and over your head and then touch your toes to the ground above your head. Repeat. *(Figure 100)*

Most beneficial to: Legs, lower back and stomach.

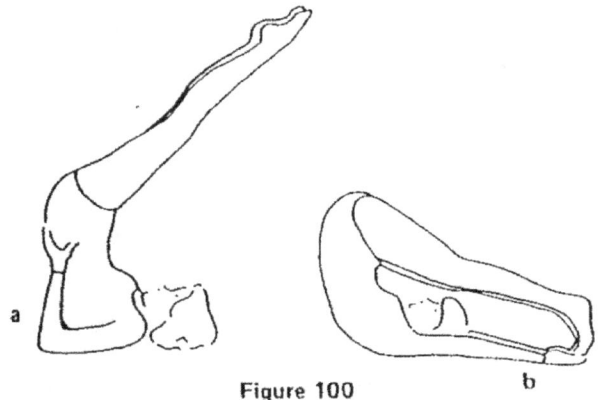

Figure 100

Leg Raiser

Sitting with your legs outstretched, lean back slightly and support yourself by putting your hands on the floor at your sides. First, lift the right leg as high as you can without bending your knees or lifting your buttocks from the floor. Alternate legs. Now lift both your legs at the same time. Lift *high.* Remember--do not bend your knees. You may have to lean back slightly more to do this.

Most beneficial to: Legs and stomach.

Leg Bounce

Sit with your hands at each side on the floor and keep your heels down. Slap your legs on the floor--first right, then left, then right, then left, etc. Then slap both legs at the same time.

Most beneficial to: Legs.

Seat Bounce

Supporting yourself with your hands on the floor at your sides, bounce your buttocks on the floor.

Most beneficial to: Buttocks.

Hold Leg Up by Foot

Sit in the V-stretch position. Now grab feet from the inside, near instep. Raise your right leg straight up; then straighten knee. Alternate legs.

Note: If the knee doesn't straighten, try taking left hand and pressing down on right knee--it may help.

Now lift both legs up in the same manner. Keep your knees straight. Try to hold this position for a few moments.

Try to find a "flat" spot when you lean back. It'll make the exercise easier. *(Figure 101)*

Most beneficial to: Legs and lower back.

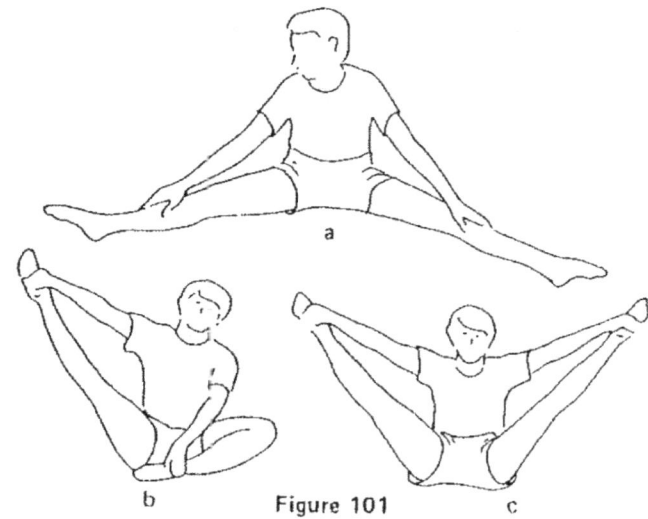

Figure 101

For the next 13 exercises, start by lying flat on your back.

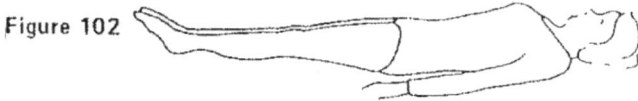

Figure 102

Roll Up to Shoulders

Lie on your back; bring your knees up. Bring your ankles to the sides and hold them with your hands. Roll up *slowly,* inch-by-inch, from the buttocks until you are high up on your shoulders. Now come down slowly, with your lower back coming down before your buttocks. This is a great stretcher for the back. *(Figure 103)*

Most beneficial to: Back.

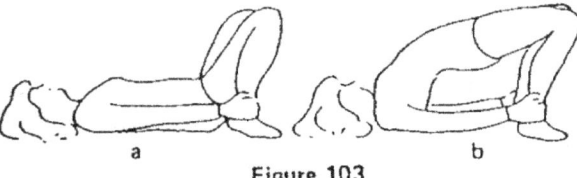

Figure 103

Roll Up Into Backbend

Lie on your back. Hold your ankles with your hands. Roll up slowly from your buttocks until you're high up on your shoulders. Put your arms over your head and push up into a backbend. Arch *high.* Now come down onto your shoulders and then down to your buttocks very *slowly.* A terrific toning exercise! *(Figure 104)*

Most beneficial to: Back.

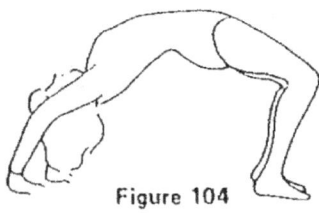

Figure 104

Each Leg Up

Lie on your back, with your knees straight. First raise your right leg high, then your left. Repeat.

Most beneficial to: Stomach and legs.

Both Legs Ups

Lie on your back, with your lower back touching the floor. With your knees straight, raise both your legs at the same time. While bringing your legs down, stretch your lower back so it continues to touch the floor. It's worth it! Repeat.

Most beneficial to: Stomach and legs.

Leg Lift

Lie on your back. The lower back should be flat on the floor, knees bent and slightly apart; shoulders down, arms stretched out, and palms upward. Bend your right knee toward chest. Bring your leg up as high as possible and straighten out the knee. Lower leg slowly until it rests on the floor, keeping your lower back flat on the floor. Now bend your knee up to the starting position. Alternate legs and repeat.

Most beneficial to: Stomach, legs and lower back.

Each Knee to Chest

Lie on your back, bend your right knee up to your chest. With hands clasped in front of your calves, pull the right knee toward your chest. Alternate knees and repeat. *(Figure 105)*

Most beneficial to: Legs.

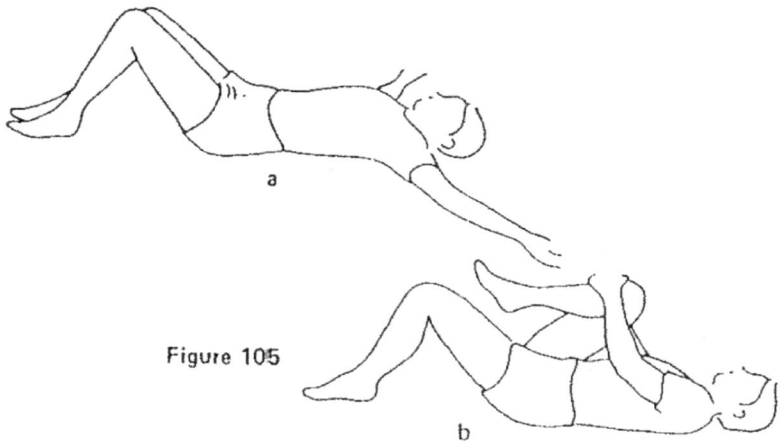

Figure 105

Both Knees to Chest

While lying on your back, with hands clasped in front of calves, bend both knees up to your chest. Pull your knees toward your chest. While bringing your legs down again, stretch your lower back so it touches the floor. Repeat.
Most beneficial to: Legs.

Legs Straight Up

Support your hips on your hands, elbows on the floor. Pointing legs upward, lift as high as you can. Keep your legs straight, with your upper back on the floor. Hold for a minute. *(Figure 106)*
Most beneficial to: Stomach and legs.

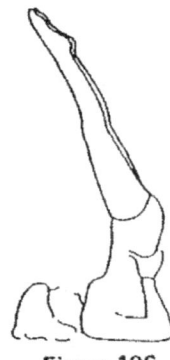

Figure 106

Bicycle

Supporting hips on hands and elbows on the floor, rotate your legs as if pedaling a bicycle. Start pedaling slowly, then faster. Rotate your legs in a circle-- this is a great firming exercise. *(Figure 107)*
Most beneficial to: Legs and stomach.

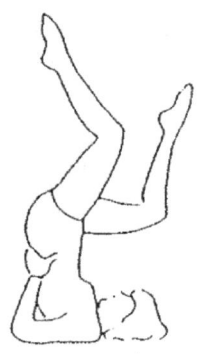

Figure 107

Figure "8"

Lie on your back, arms outstretched at the sides, palms turned up. Draw your knees to your chest. Keep your knees together and arms on the floor. Now drop both knees (together) to the right until they touch the floor. Draw them up towards your right elbow. Hold for a few moments. Now put knees back over your chest. Hold again. Then drop your knees to the left side (together) and then up to your left elbow. Bring your legs back to the starting position. Each side makes a loop of the "8." *(Figure 108)*

Most beneficial to: Thighs, legs and stomach

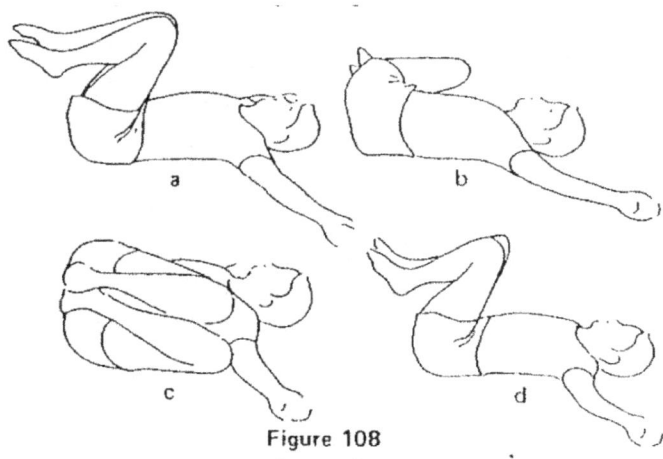

Figure 108

"I"

Lying on the floor, draw your knees up to your chest and extend your arms out from the shoulders. Now raise your legs straight up--knees straight. Then bend your knees slightly, spread your legs and turn your toes out. Draw your knees back to your chest and repeat exercise. *(Figure 109)*

Most beneficial to: Legs and stomach.

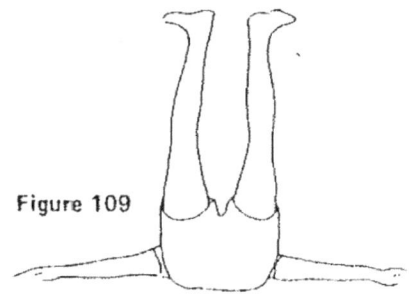

Figure 109

Spine Rock

Sit with your knees up and bent, cross your feet. Now grasp your feet with your hands. Then rock back onto your shoulders. Rock from side to side on your shoulders, then up to a sitting position and forward, touching forehead on floor in front of your feet. As you are rocking back into the sitting position, stretch your lower back so that it touches the floor on your way up. This is a great spine stretcher. *(Figure 110)*

Most beneficial to: Lower back, stomach and legs.

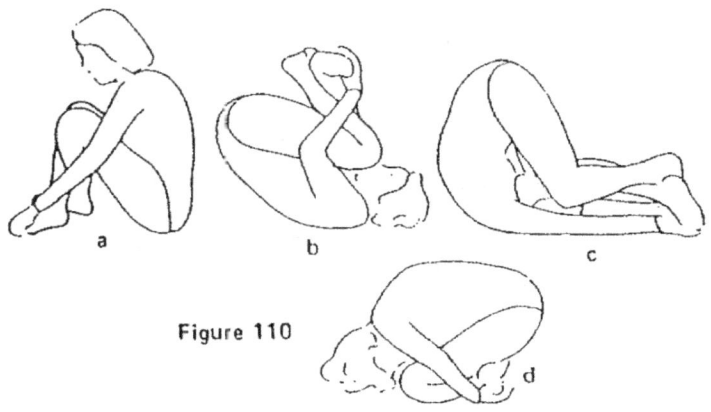

Figure 110

Plough

Lie on your back with arms stretched straight up over your head. Now roll up onto your shoulders, bringing your feet over your head. Hold your feet with your hands and move them apart and then together (about 6 inches). Repeat. *(Figure 111)*

Most beneficial to: Back, legs and arms.

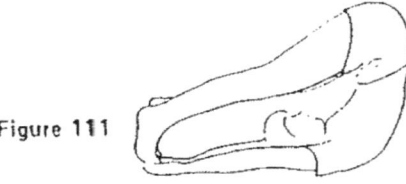

Figure 111

Shoulder Balance

Roll up onto your shoulders and bring your legs straight up. Do not bend your knees. Put your hands up on each side of your legs. Balance for a few moments.
Most beneficial to: Legs and stomach

For the next four exercises, we will begin by lying flat on our stomachs.

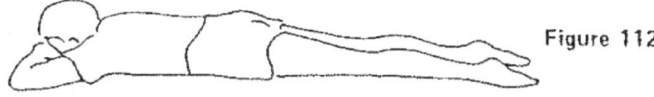
Figure 112

Lift Each Leg, Then Both

Support your chin in your hands. Lift your right leg behind you, keeping your hips on the floor. Do the same with the left leg, keeping knees straight. Now lift both your legs at the same time. *(Figure 113)*
Most beneficial to: Legs and stomach.

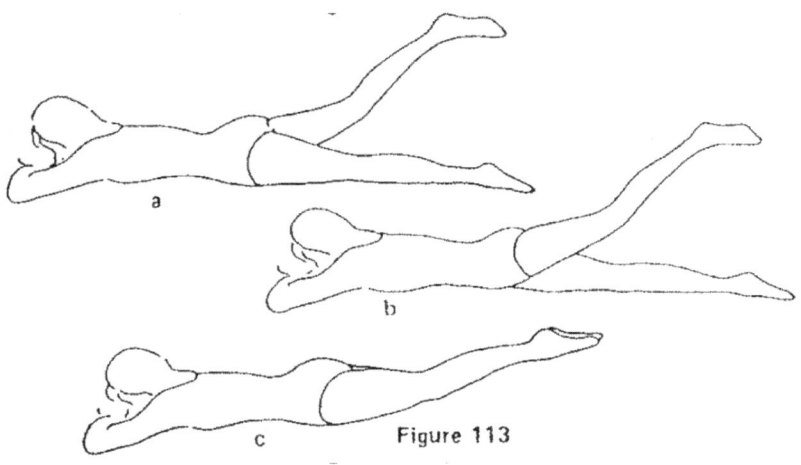
Figure 113

Half Push Ups

Put your hands palms down, on the floor in front of your shoulders. Lift both your legs off the floor behind you, as high as you can. Do not bend your knees or lift hips off the floor. Push up with your hands, lifting your chest off the floor. Then, come back down to the floor, with elbows first, then chest, then chin.
Most beneficial to: Stomach.

Push Up

Put your hands flat on the floor alongside your shoulders, fingers pointing forward. Raise your body keeping your back and legs straight, and feet on the floor. Straighten arms. Now lower your body until your chest is about an inch or two from the floor. Repeat.
Most beneficial to: Back, arms and legs.

Push Up to Inverted "V"

Lying on the floor, raise your chest slightly. Put your hands closer to your shoulders. Push up with hands and "walk" into an "Inverted V." Keep your hands on the floor and stay up on your toes--do not drop your heels! Then walk back down--first drop hips, then elbows, then chest and then chin--in that order. Smile, it's working as you do it! *(Figure 114)*

   Most beneficial to: Lower back, arms and legs.

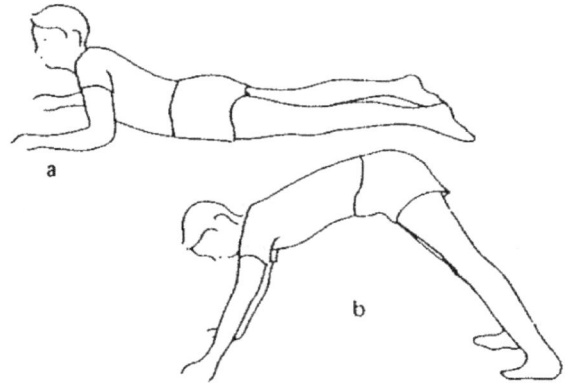

Figure 114

For the next six exercises, sit on your feet. Keep your back straight.

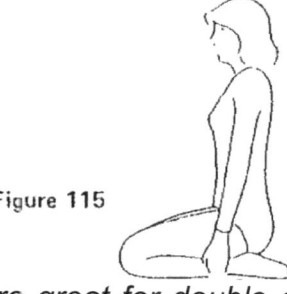

Figure 115

   The first three exercises are great for double chins and stiff necks. The last three are good for stiff shoulders or upper back.
   For the shoulder stretchers, let your shoulders do the moving, and elbows hang limp.

Neck Fore and Aft
   Pull your neck forward as if trying to pull your chin to your chest. Then pull it way back. Your head should go back far enough to feel the stretch through the front of your neck. *(Figure 116)*
   Most beneficial to: Neck.

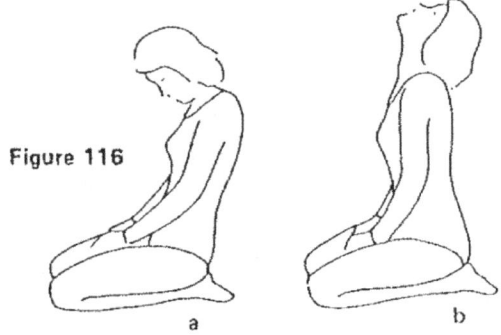

Figure 116

a   b

Neck to Side

Move your neck first to the right side and then to the left side. Repeat. You should feel it pull.

Most beneficial to: Neck.

Full Neck Circle

Move your head forward, then to the right, then to the back, to the left and forward again, making a circle. Try to move smoothly without moving your shoulders. Repeat. This is great for relaxing, too.

Most beneficial to: Neck.

Shoulders Up and Down

Keeping everything but your shoulders still, bring them up as high as possible, as if to touch your ears. Then drop your shoulders as far as possible. Feel the pull?. Repeat.

Most beneficial to: Shoulders.

Shoulders Fore and Aft

Bring shoulders forward as far as possible. Then push them way back.

Most beneficial to: Shoulders.

Shoulder Circles

Move both shoulders up high, then back, then down, and then forward, making a circle. Now do it a little faster and more smoothly. Next, reverse the circle--down, back, up and forward. Now, start the circle with the right shoulder by bringing it back. Keep rotating it in a circle and start the left one at the same time. The left one will be one step behind the right. Now reverse, with the left shoulder leading.

Most beneficial to: Shoulders.

Raise Each Leg

Lie on your left side. Support your head with your left hand, elbow on the floor. Raise your right arm straight up from the shoulder. Raise your right leg up to touch your right hand. Alternate on the right side with the left leg. This is great for toning! Work up to 50 times with each leg. *(Figure 117)*

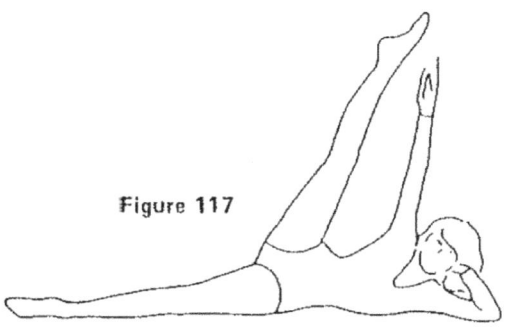

Figure 117

Most beneficial to: Legs, waist and buttocks.

For the next three, we will get down on all fours. Put your hands below shoulders--fingers pointed halfway to the outside.

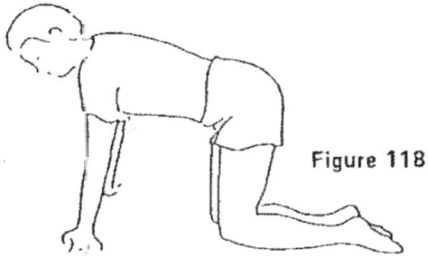

Figure 118

Back Pick Up and Drop

Raise your back as high and rounded as you can. Then lower your back to a "concave" position. Repeat.

Most beneficial to: Back.

Extend Leg and Rotate

Extend your right leg straight from the hip. Bring your knee back, but do not set it on the floor--hold it a couple of inches above. Extend the leg twice more. Now rotate the leg, keeping it straight. Repeat, making a larger circle. Alternate sides and repeat with the left leg. This is a terrific trimming exercise for the thighs. *(Figure 119)*

Most beneficial to: Thighs and legs.

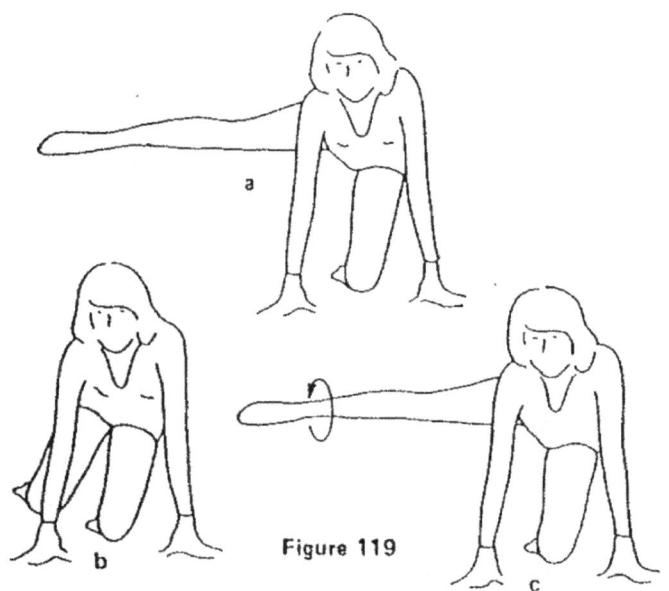

Figure 119

Knees to Elbow

Still on all fours, bring your right knee up to your right elbow. Repeat three times. Alternate sides and repeat.

Most beneficial to: Thighs and legs.

The next four will be in the straight kneel position. Bend from the waist only, unless otherwise indicated. Hips should stay still. Keep head forward and up.

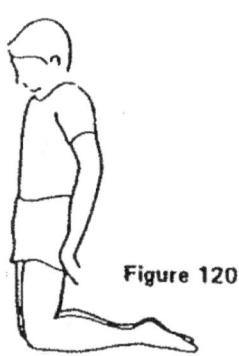

Figure 120

Sit Down to Feet

Kneel straight up. Arch back; stomach and chest out. Now lower yourself to sit on your feet, shoulders forward and your back arched. Then rise up to a straight kneel. *(Figure 121)*

Most beneficial to: Legs and back.

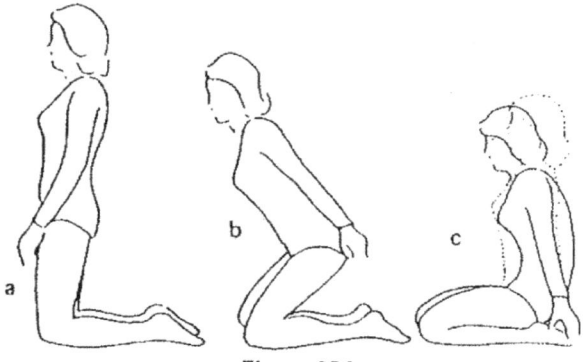

Figure 121

Sit Down to Feet/Chest to Knees

Move from kneeling straight up to sitting on your feet. Lean forward from your waist and bring your chest to your knees. Keep your back straight. Rise up to a straight kneel. *(Figure 122)*

Most beneficial to: Legs and back.

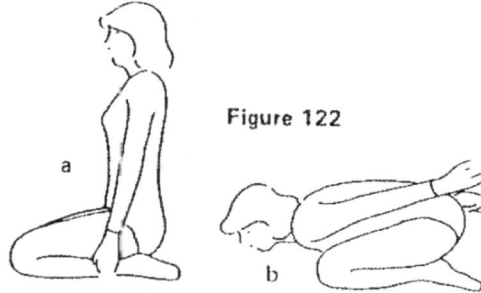

Figure 122

Kneeling Tilt Back

Still kneeling, hold body straight and stiff. Now tilt back, tightening your buttocks and extending your arms in front for balance. Hold for a few seconds. Repeat.

Most beneficial to: Legs and stomach.

Buttocks Bounce

From the kneeling position, sit on the floor and hold your ankles alongside your legs. Now, bounce your buttocks on the floor between your feet. *(Figure 123)*

Most beneficial to: Legs.

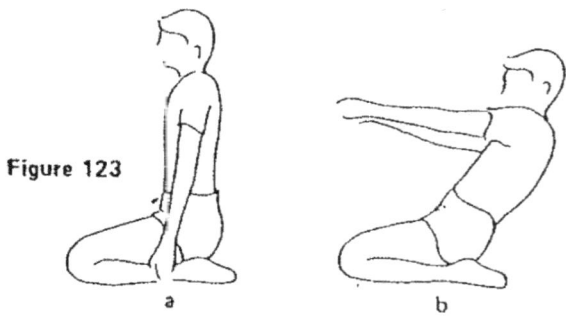

Figure 123

Rise to Side

Sitting with your hands on your ankles and your ankles alongside your legs, raise up and out to the right, holding the right ankle only. Sit back down and do the same, holding the left ankle. Repeat. *(Figure 124)*

Most beneficial to: Thighs.

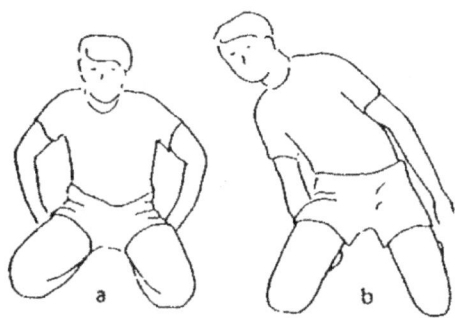

Figure 124

Touch Feet

From a kneeling position, bend back from the waist and touch your right foot with your right hand; then your left foot with your left hand. *(Figure 125)*

Most beneficial to: Legs, stomach and back.

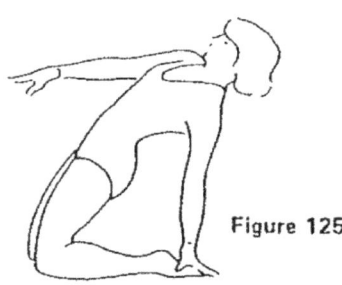

Figure 125

Touch Between Feet

Again, on your knees, bend back and touch the floor with your right hand. Come up to a straight kneel, then do the same with your left hand. *(Figure 126)*

Most beneficial to: Legs, stomach and back.

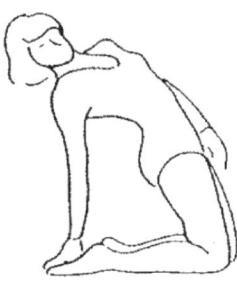

Figure 126

Fish

In the kneeling position, lean back and hold your feet or ankles with your hands. Drop to your elbows and come back up. This exercise is really great for toning the whole torso! *(Figure 127)*

Most beneficial to: Legs, stomach and back.

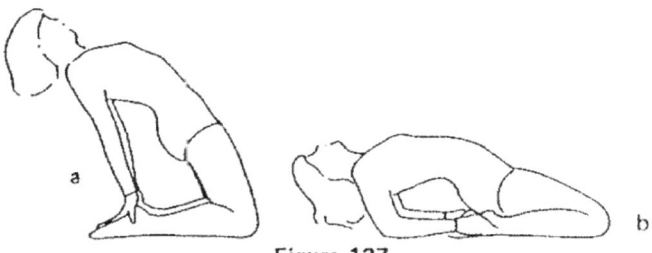

Figure 127

Look Mom--No Hands!

While kneeling, extend arms straight out in front of you. Now, lean back until you are about four inches from the floor. Be sure to arch your back and hold your hips up from your feet. Now come up to a straight kneel. *(Figure 128)*

Do this exercise *slowly* and to avoid hitting your head, use padding. These exercises are great for your thighs. You'll see the difference in no time.

Most beneficial to: Legs, stomach and back.

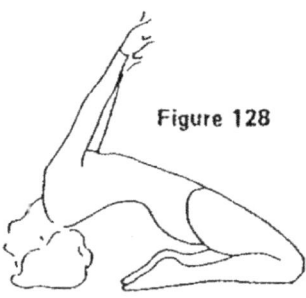

Figure 128

Stand up and "shake out" your leg; let the muscles relax a bit. For the next five, we will be on our feet.

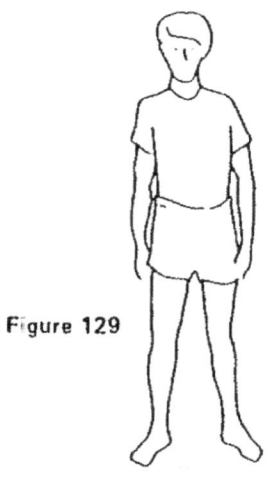

Figure 129

Arm Pulleys

With your feet flat on the floor, reach up high with your right arm, fingers pointed up. At the same time, pull down with your left arm, fingers pointing down. You should be pulling in opposite directions. Alternate; left arm up, right arm down. Repeat.

Most beneficial to: Sides and arms.

Arm Swing

Keeping feet flat on the floor and facing forward, put your right arm straight back and left arm straight forward. Now turn and twist from the waist, so that the left arm is straight back and right arm is straight forward. Keep elbows straight. Repeat. *(Figure 130)*

Most beneficial to: Waist and arms.

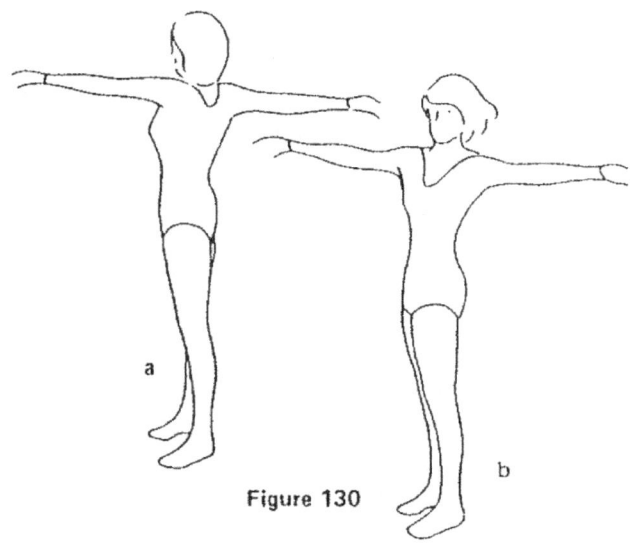

Figure 130

Jumping Jacks

Stand with your feet together and arms at your sides. Jump and stretch your legs apart while raising your arms and clap hands over head. Jump back to your starting position. Repeat. Now do it faster. *(Figure 131)*

Most beneficial to: Legs and arms.

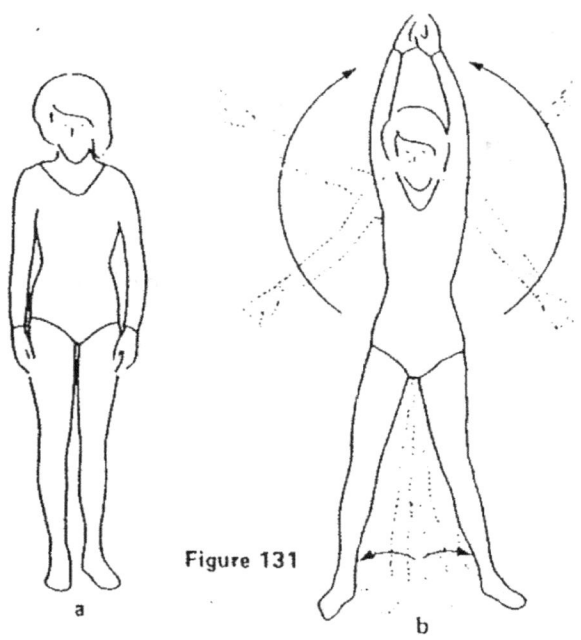

Figure 131

Run in Place

Raising each foot at least five inches off the floor, jog in place. Start slowly and quicken the pace.

Most beneficial to: Legs.

Look Mom--No Rope!

Hold an imaginary jump rope in your hands. Imagine swinging it. When the rope hits the floor, jump over it--one foot in front of the other. Alternate feet. Now try both feet over at the same time.

Most beneficial to: The whole body!

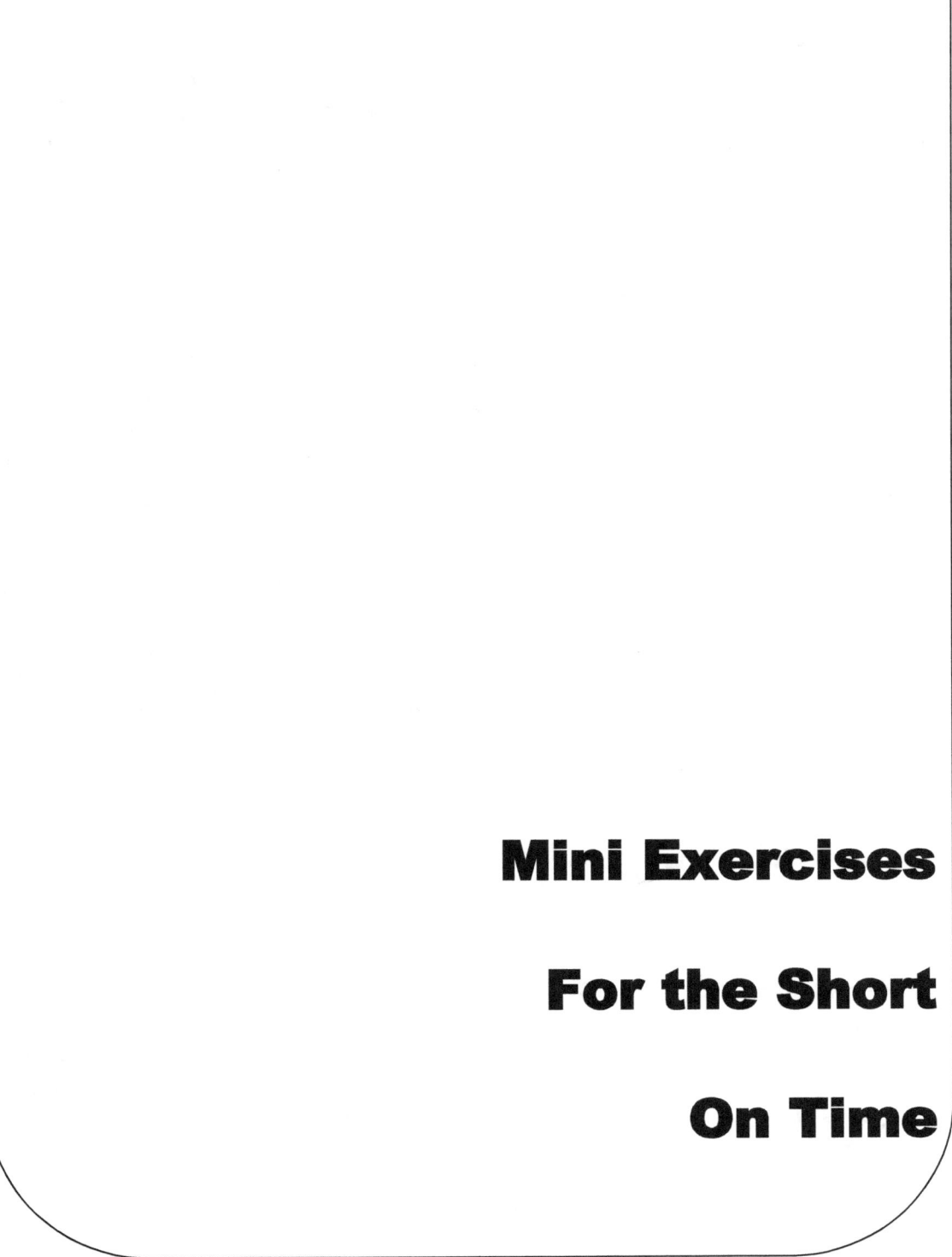

Mini Exercises

For the Short

On Time

(A Crash Course....)

Spine to Floor

Lie on your back with legs extended. Push your spine (from the top to the bottom) flat down to the floor. Keep your heels and legs on the floor. Lift hips upward, but do not lift up buttocks. Try to put your hands between your lower spine and the floor. You should not be able to get them between if you are doing the exercise correctly. *(Figure 132)*

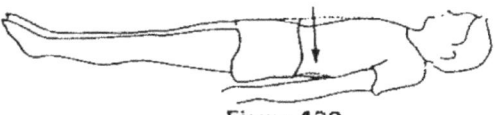

Figure 132

It may be impossible to get your spine all the way down to the floor with the first few tries, but it will get easier each time.

This exercise is particularly good for people with lower back problems. Starting the exercise program with this stretcher will help in the following exercises.

Most beneficial to: Lower back.

Neck to Floor

Lie on your back with legs extended. Push the back of your neck flat down to the floor. Do this by pulling your chin down toward your chest; without lifting your head from the floor. You will not be able to get your fingers underneath your neck if you are doing this correctly. *(Figure 133)*

If you can't do it correctly right away, keep trying!

Most beneficial to: Neck.

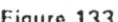

Figure 133

Before starting these next four exercises, let's warm up by sitting with the soles of your feet together. Now hold your feet with your hands. Bring your heels toward you and lean forward at the same time. As you are doing this, try to pull your knees downward without using your hands. Repeat.

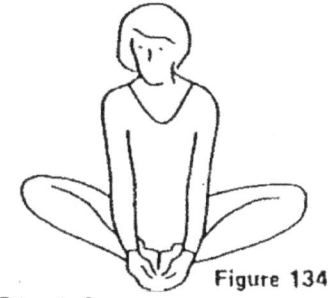

Figure 134

Soles Together Overhead Stretch

First, with your right hand, stretch upward while keeping your left hand on your left knee. Stretch as high as you can. Now do the same with the left hand, putting your right hand on your right knee. *(Figure 135)*

Most beneficial to: Thighs and waist.

Figure 135

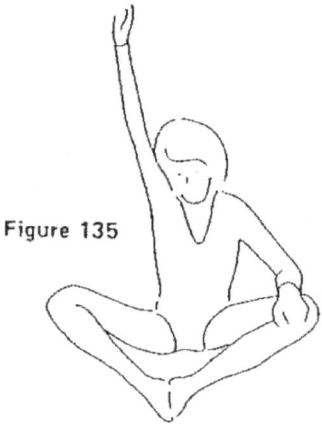

Soles Together Overhead Stretch/Wrist

Stretch up with your right arm. With the left hand, hold your right wrist and pull down toward your head, leaning slightly to the left. Then alternate sides--stretch up with your left arm, right hand holding left wrist and pull while leaning slightly to the right. Repeat. *(Figure 136)*

Most beneficial to: Thighs, waist and arms.

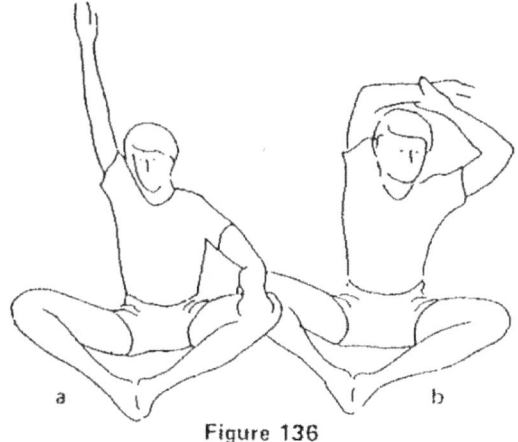

a   b

Figure 136

Soles Together Overhead Side Stretch

Reach up and over your head with right arm. Rest your left hand on your feet and lean to the left just enough to feel a slight pull. Now repeat with the left hand overhead and the right hand on your feet. Repeat. *(Figure 137)*

Most beneficial to: Thighs and waist.

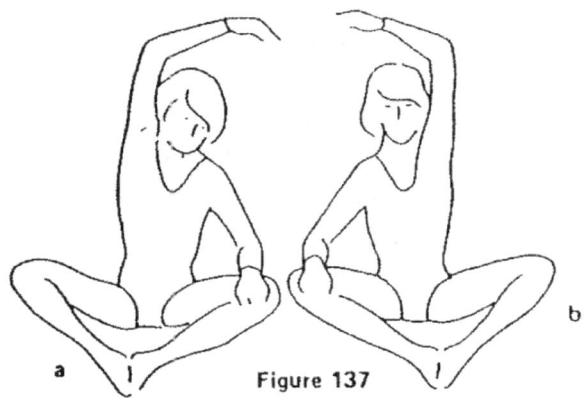

Figure 137

Soles Together Head to Feet

Still sitting with the soles of your feet together, hold your feet with both hands. Bend forward and *stretch* until your head touches your feet. Do not lift your buttocks from the floor. *(Figure 138)*

Most beneficial to: Thighs and back.

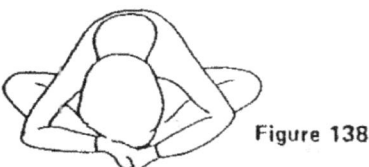

Figure 138

Now stand with your feet flat on the floor, feet spread shoulder width apart and knees straight.

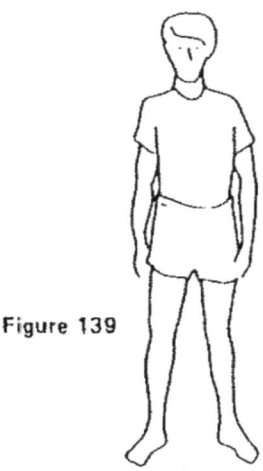

Figure 139

Regular Toe Touch

Touch your toes with the tips of your fingers, keeping your legs straight. *Stretch* up, reaching as high as possible. Repeat. *(Figure 140)*
   Most beneficial to: Legs, back and stomach.

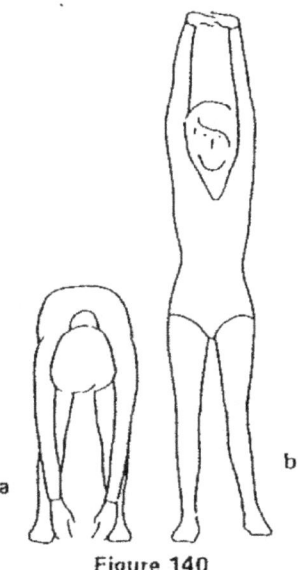

Figure 140

Toe Touch/Hands to Floor
   Touch the floor with the palms of your hands. Keep your knees straight. Stretch way up with your arms, hands upward. Repeat. *(Figure 141)*
   Most beneficial to: Legs, back and stomach.

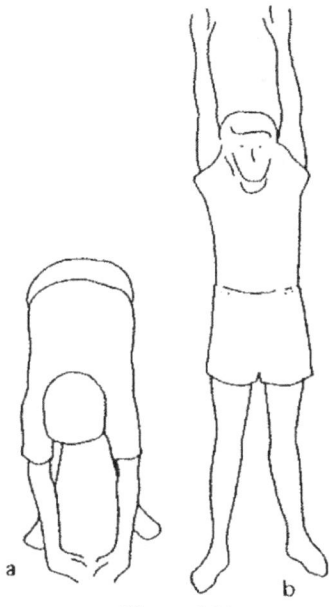

Figure 141

Fan Toe Touch
   Stand with your feet spread shoulder width apart and your arms outstretched. With your right hand, touch your left toes with the tips of your fingers. Come up

85

and stretch with your arms up high. Alternate--your left hand to your right toes. Keep your knees straight! *(Figure 142)*

Most beneficial to: Legs, back and stomach.

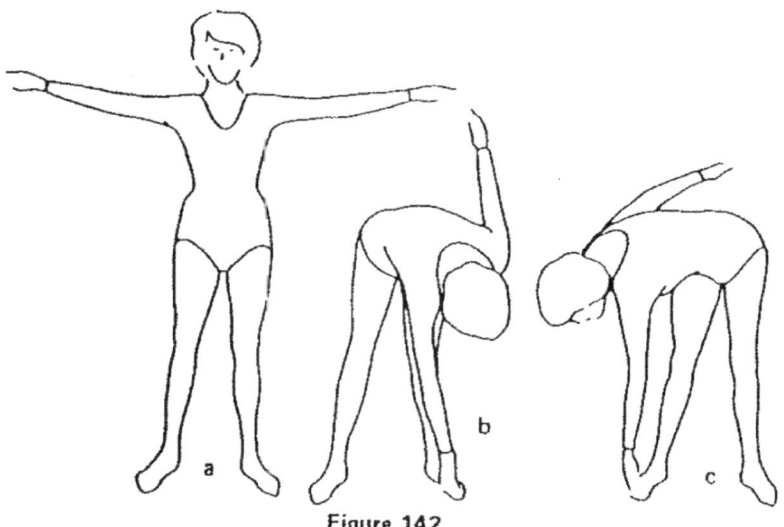

Figure 142

Knee Bend

Hold your arms straight out. Bend your knees and go down into a "squatting" position with your feet flat on the floor. Then stand up straight. *(Figure 143)*

Most beneficial to: Legs and lower back.

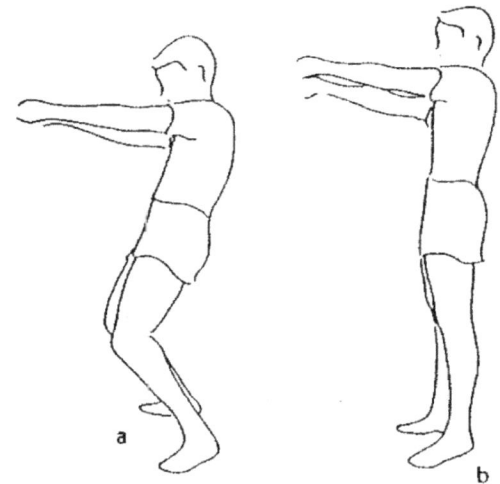

Figure 143

For the next three exercises, sit on the floor with your legs stretched out in a "V" position. Keep your legs stretched as far apart as possible for the best results.

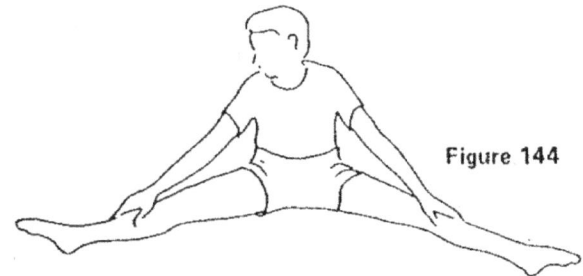

Figure 144

Hands to Toes

Sitting in the V-position, touch your right hand to your right foot, with your left hand resting at your side. Alternate and touch your left hand to your left foot. Repeat. *(Figure 145)*

Most beneficial to: Thighs.

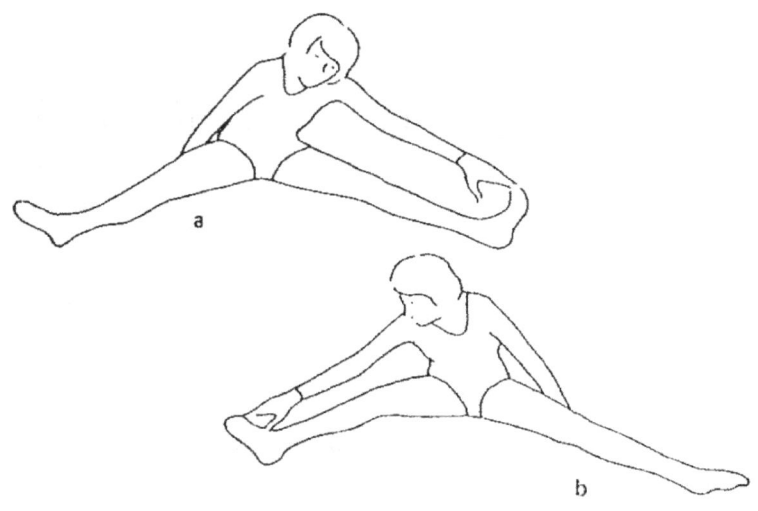

a

b

Figure 145

Toe to Toe Swing

With arms extended together, point your fingers forward and swing your arms from right foot to left foot. Keep your arms in a straight line and your body forward. *(Figure 146)*

Most beneficial to: Thighs.

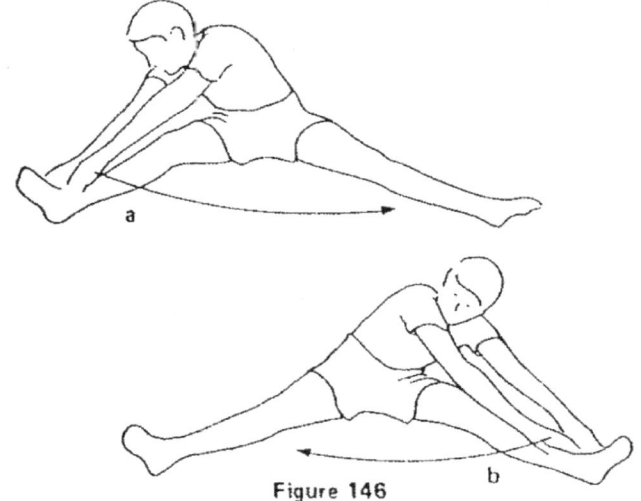

Figure 146

Head to Knees

Sitting in the V-stretch position, lean over and touch your forehead to your right knee. Alternate and touch your forehead to your left knee. *(Figure 147)*

Most beneficial to: Thighs and back.

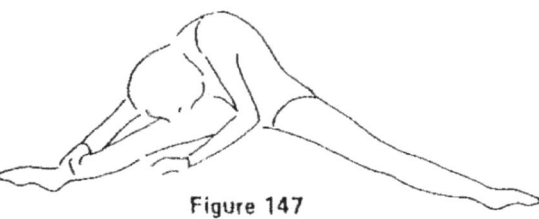

Figure 147

For the next three exercises, start by sitting with legs stretched forward and knees straight.

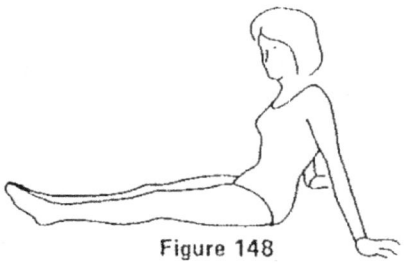

Figure 148

Lean Forward/Head to Knees

Sit with your legs outstretched and your toes pointed forward. Bend forward, bringing your head to your knees. Let your arms move forward. Do not bend your knees. You'll feel pulling in your legs, particularly behind knees. *(Figure 149)*

Most beneficial to: Legs and back.

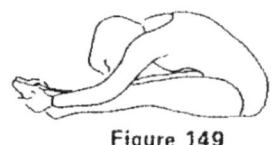

Figure 149

Sit Ups

Lie back with your arms extended overhead. Sit up and touch your toes with your hands. Keep your knees straight and your heels on the floor. *(Figure 150)*
Most beneficial to: Stomach and back.

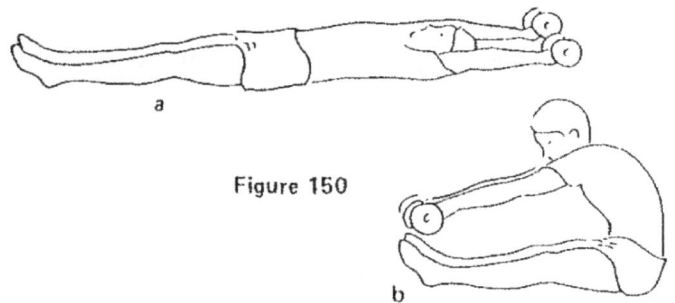

Figure 150

Leg Raiser

Sitting with your legs extended, lean back slightly and support yourself with your hands at your sides. First lift the right leg as high as you can, keeping knees straight, and buttocks on the floor. Then the left leg. Now lift both legs at the same time. Lift *high.* Do not bend knees. *(Figure 151)*
Most beneficial to: Legs and stomach.

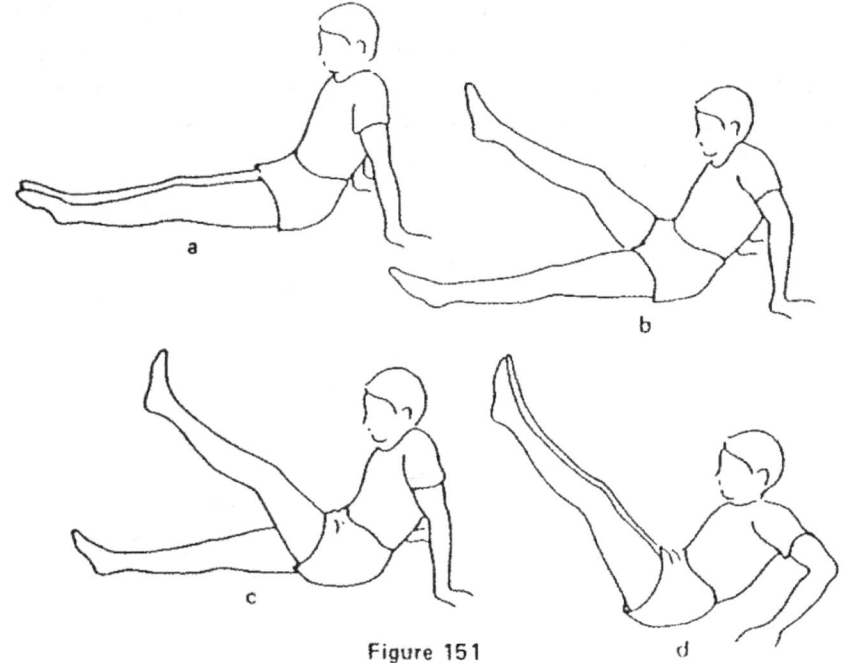

Figure 151

Start the next two exercises by lying flat on your stomach.

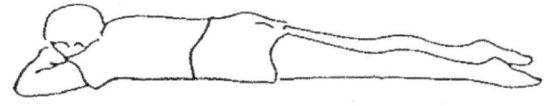

Figure 152

Half Push Ups

Put hands palm side down, on the floor in front of your shoulders. Lift both legs at the same time off the floor, as high as you can. Again, keep your knees straight and your hips on the floor. Push up with your hands, lifting your chest off the floor. Then lower yourself back to the floor with your elbows first, then your chest and then your chin. *(Figure 153)*

Most beneficial to: Stomach.

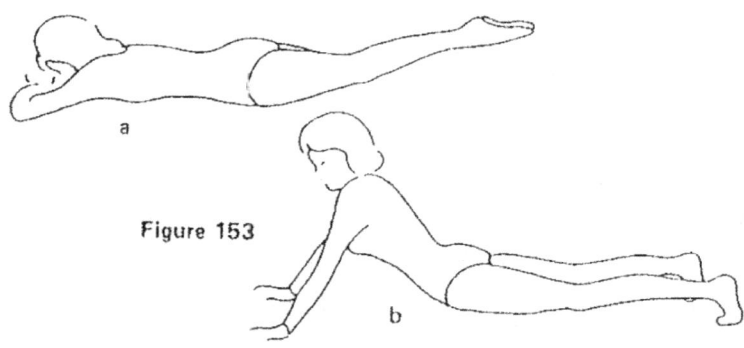

Figure 153

Push Ups

Lying on your stomach, put your hands flat on the floor alongside your shoulders, fingers pointing forward. Raise your body, keeping back and legs straight, and feet on the floor. Straighten arms. Now lower your body until chest is about an inch or two from the floor. Repeat. *(Figure 154)*

Most beneficial to: Back, arms and legs.

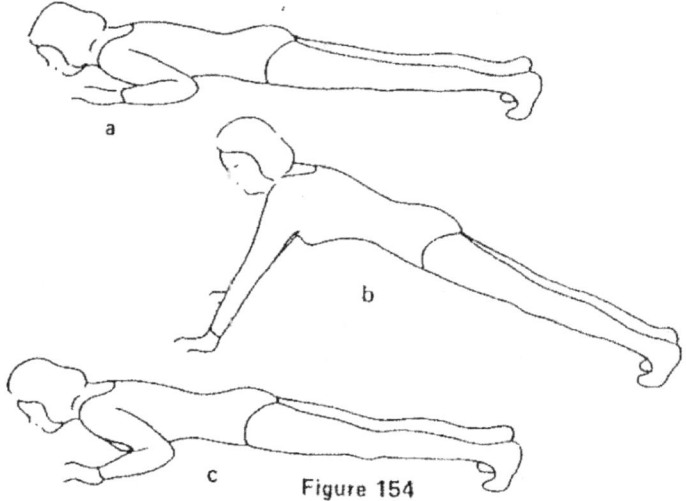

Figure 154

Run in Place

Standing, raise each foot at least five inches off the floor and jog in place. Start slowly and go faster. *(Figure 155)*

Most beneficial to: Legs.

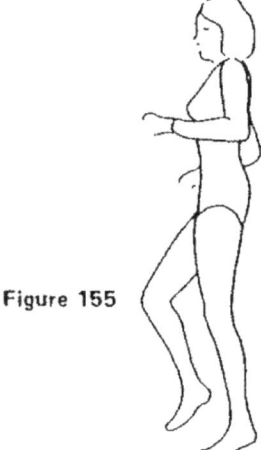

Figure 155

These exercises can be substituted with any combination. But be sure to use a few from each starting position and for each part of your body.

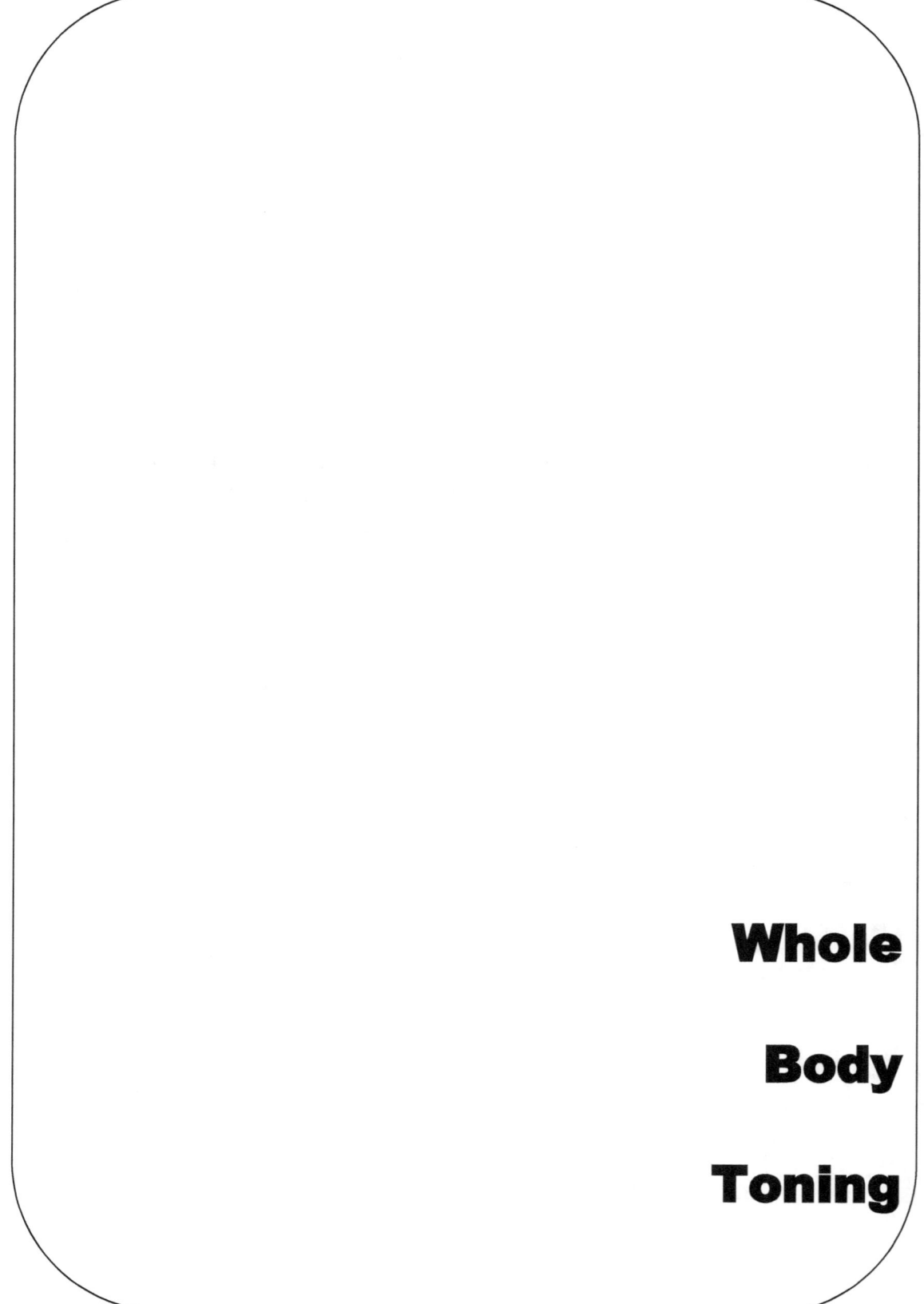

Whole

Body

Toning

(Jumping...Jogging...Lifting)

JUMP ROPE

It's best to jump rope wearing either running shoes or sneakers, since it is important to land on the balls of your feet. Be sure to wear clothing, such as a sweatsuit or leotards, that won't catch the rope.

Although my favorite jump rope is a professional one, a piece of clothesline with knotted ends will suffice. To determine the proper length, hold the rope with an end in each hand--the rope should reach the floor from chest level.

Breathe only through your nose while you jump. If you breathe through your mouth, you get out of breath easier. Jump lightly, landing on the balls of your feet. Rotate the rope with your wrists only, moving your arms as little as possible.

Time yourself while you jump. Although you may only be able to jump a few minutes at first, try to work up to 15 minutes. It's an invigorating exercise!

If you have a heart condition, do not jump rope unless you have your doctor's approval.

Here are seven jumps to try:
1) Jump with both feet over the rope at the same time.
2) Right foot over rope first.
3) Left foot over rope first.
4) While holding your rope still, start jogging, lifting your feet about six inches off the floor. Now start rotating the rope as you jog. Jump over at the count of four. The first jump will be with the right foot, step with the left foot; step with the right foot, then jump over with the left foot. Then start with the left foot and repeat.
5) Cross your hands when rope is up. Jump. Then uncross hands. *(Figure 156)*

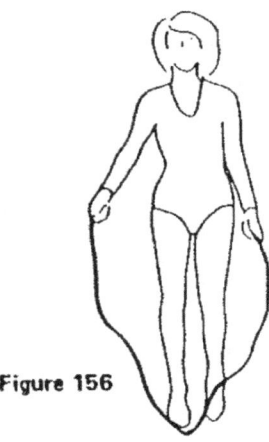

Figure 156

6) Jump over rope sideways. *(Figure 157)*

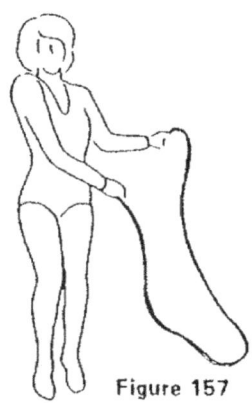

Figure 157

7) Jump backwards over rope.
Most beneficial to: The Whole Body!

JOGGING
(Great for the Body--and the Mind!)

Wear loose comfortable clothing. jogging suits are not essential, but are practical. Dress seasonably. Be especially cautious in the summer so heat exhaustion does not occur. Running shoes with good arch supports are best: avoid thin-soled tennis shoes. Heavy socks are good not only for absorbency but keep shoes from rubbing against your feet.

Jog with your back straight and your head up. Hold arms a few inches away from your body, with your elbows bent. Try to land on your heels and roll forward onto the balls of your feet. If this is difficult, try landing on the "flats" of your feet. Landing on the balls of the feet can cause soreness in the legs, especially if you're not in good physical shape. Keep your strides short, and breath deeply with your mouth slightly open.

The best place to jog is a running track, but that's not always possible. Running on grass is good to start on.

If you get tired, stop and walk, but walk at a fast pace. Increase your running time each time you're out. A regular schedule is best.

Most beneficial to: The Whole Body!

WEIGHT LIFTING
(Take the Weight Off Your Shoulders!)

Since building muscles is not always desirable, I have included these five weight lifting exercises that will not promote great muscle building.

Begin by using three-pound ladies' dumbbells or five-pound men's dumbbells. If you're feeling really ambitious, use dumbbells with interchangeable weights. Begin with the lighter weights and add on.

Half Sit-Ups

With one weight in each hand, lie back with your arms stretched overhead. Sit up and touch your toes with the weights. Be careful not to drop the weights on your feet! Keep your knees straight and your heels on the floor. It will be easier to keep your feet on the floor if you point your toes forward.

Most beneficial to: Stomach, back and legs.

Toe Touch

Standing with one weight in each hand, touch the floor in front of your feet with the weights. Keep your knees straight. *Stretch* up, reaching as high as possible. Repeat. *(Figure 158)*

Most beneficial to: Legs, back and stomach.

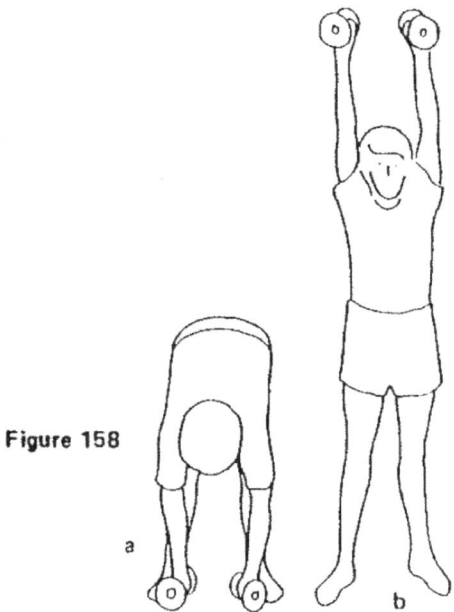

Figure 158

Arm Pulleys

Standing with a weight in each hand, and feet flat on the floor, reach up *high* with your right arm and pull down with your left arm. You're pulling in opposite directions. Now reverse--left arm is up and right arm is down. Repeat.

Most beneficial to: Waist and arms.

Arm Swing

Stand with weights in each hand, keep your feet flat on the floor and face forward. Put your right arm straight back and your left arm straight forward. Now turn and twist from the waist, so that the left arm is straight back and the right arm is straight forward. Keep your elbows straight. Repeat.

Most beneficial to: Waist and arms.

These exercises have been described earlier in the book but without the use of weights. With the weights you will feel more pulling and, you'll benefit more. They're really beneficial for people who have done sit-ups and toe touches for years, to increase the effect.